Clinical Education
in the Health Professions

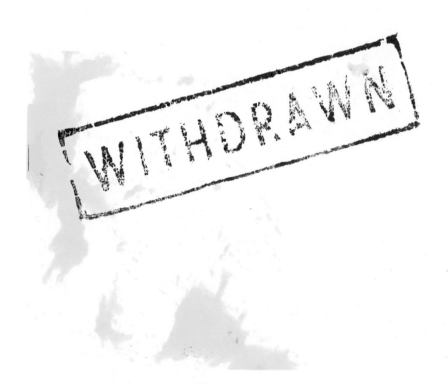

D1341339

Clinical Education
in the Health Professions

Edited by · **Clare Delany** · **Elizabeth Molloy**

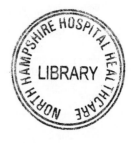

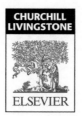

CHURCHILL LIVINGSTONE

ELSEVIER

Sydney   Edinburgh   London   New York   Philadelphia   St Louis   Toronto

Churchill Livingstone
is an imprint of Elsevier

Elsevier Australia. ACN 001 002 357
(a division of Reed International Books Australia Pty Ltd)
Tower 1, 475 Victoria Avenue, Chatswood, NSW 2067

ELSEVIER

National Library of Australia Cataloguing-in-Publication Data

_____

Clinical education in the health professions / edited by
        Clare Delany and Elizabeth Molloy.

ISBN: 978 0 7295 3900 5 (pbk.)

Includes index.
Bibliography.

Medicine--Study and teaching.

Delany, Clare.
Molloy, Elizabeth.

610.7

_____

Publishing Editor: Sunalie Silva
Developmental Editor: Meg O'Hanlon
Publishing Services Manager: Helena Klijn
Editorial Coordinator: Lauren Allsop
Edited by Brenda Hamilton
Proofread and indexed by Forsyth Publishing Services
Cover and internal design by Avril Makula
Typeset by TNQ Books and Journals Pvt Ltd
Printed in China by China Translation and Printing Services

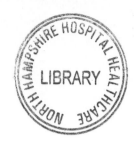

Contents

Preface

We shall not cease from our exploration
And the end of all our exploring
Will be to arrive where we started
And know the place for the first time
TS Eliot

There were two bicycles, two people and two key ideas that prompted the genesis of this book. In March 2007, we (the editors) were training for a bike ride along the Great Ocean Road, Victoria. At the time, we had been preparing a curriculum support package for clinical educators in a newly developed undergraduate physiotherapy program. We decided there was a need to produce a book that addressed the complexity of teaching and learning in the clinical education environment. The two related ideas that underpin the book were a need to make the theories and evidence that guide teaching and learning in clinical education more explicit; and a need to promote increased agency in both clinical educators and students in their respective roles as teachers and learners.

Throughout the book, the role of the clinical educator is recognised and promoted as one that empowers students to be active, engaged and mature learners. Our underlying premise is that if clinicians focus on how to best facilitate learning in their students, then their teaching preparation will be directed towards the needs of the learner rather than following prescriptive methods of teaching based on their past experience as students and/or teachers.

We found theories about adult learning to be the most useful and relevant to inform the writing of this book. By increasing the transparency of educational theory, we hope that clinical educators will develop their own teaching methods and styles from a secure theoretical platform that provides relevant principles, direction and support. With a background of empirical evidence and explanatory theoretical frameworks, educators should be more confident to approach student learning challenges using their underpinning knowledge of education, rather than requiring advice or a protocol on how to approach each individual student with a particular learning need.

Our two key ideas of highlighting theory and promoting agency are reflected throughout this book, and we would like to thank the authors for their contributions and enthusiasm in embracing these ideas in their writing about different areas of clinical education. Our intention throughout the planning and writing of this book is that the suggestions offered and, most importantly, the questions raised within each chapter of the book will encourage clinical educators and others involved in providing and thinking about clinical education to 'arrive at a place where they started and know the place for the first time'.

Editors

Dr Clare Delany is a Senior Lecturer in ethics, law and qualitative research methods at the School of Physiotherapy, The University of Melbourne, and a Clinical Ethics Fellow at the Children's Bioethics Centre at the Royal Children's Hospital in Melbourne. Clare has masters degrees in Health and Medical Law, and Physiotherapy (Manipulation). Her PhD and ongoing research interests include legal and ethical obligations of health practitioners, the role of critical reflection in clinical ethics education, healthcare communication, and ways of implementing ethical theory into clinical practice.

Dr Elizabeth Molloy is a Senior Lecturer at the Centre for Medical and Health Sciences Education at Monash University. Elizabeth teaches in the masters degree and the graduate certificate in Health Professional Education with a particular interest in the role of practitioners and university-based educators in facilitating active student learning. Elizabeth completed her PhD at The University of Melbourne in the area of feedback in clinical education, and helped to develop the physiotherapy clinical education program at Monash University. Her areas of research interest include feedback, reflective practice, and professional transitions. In addition to her work in health professional education and research, Elizabeth is a practising physiotherapist and has worked as team physiotherapist with Australian athletics teams over the last 7 years.

Contributors

Dr Rola Ajjawi is a Lecturer at the Office of Postgraduate Medical Education at The University of Sydney. She trained and worked as a physiotherapist before moving into clinical education. In her PhD she explored how experienced clinicians learnt to make decisions and to communicate these decisions with patients and students. She is about to complete postdoctoral research analysing the learning needs of GP registrars for quality prescribing, along with the design and delivery of tailored educational packages. Her research interests include developing clinical reasoning capability, workplace learning, and learning and teaching across the continuum of health professional education. In her current role, Rola is also involved in curriculum design and delivery in the Master of Medical Education Program and is leading the curriculum review process. She has published several journal articles and is co-editor of *Communicating in the Health Sciences.*

Associate Professor Anna Chur-Hansen is Deputy Head of the Discipline of Psychiatry at The University of Adelaide. Anna is a Registered Psychologist and since 2003 has held the Chair of the Australian Psychological Society's College of Health Psychologists in South Australia. Her research interests are in Medical Education (the area of her doctoral dissertation), as well as broader health professional education and interdisciplinary approaches. Anna also conducts research into patients' experiences of their healthcare and perceptions of their health and illness, along with studies on the relationship between companion animals and psychological and physical health. She loves teaching and learning, and her two West Highland White Terriers.

Megan Dalton is a Senior Lecturer Clinical Education and Convenor of the Masters of Physiotherapy Program in the School of Physiotherapy and Exercise Science at Griffith University, Queensland. She has 20 years' experience in overseeing the development of clinical education programs now at Griffith University and previously at The University of Queensland. In the last 7 years Megan has been involved in the establishment of two new physiotherapy programs, including planning, implementation and evaluation of clinical placements, and writing of the curriculum and documentation for accreditation of both programs. Megan is currently enrolled in a PhD investigating the assessment of clinical competence.

Associate Professor Megan Davidson is Head of the School of Physiotherapy at La Trobe University, Melbourne. Megan has a particular interest in clinical education having been Clinical Coordinator of the La Trobe physiotherapy program and a member of the multidisciplinary, trans-university Foundation for Quality Supervision. Her research interests in education are in the areas of interprofessional education, assessment of clinical performance, and evidence-based practice. Megan was a member of a project team funded by the Department of Human Services in 2006–07 to develop models of interprofessional clinical education. In 2007–08 she was involved in a project funded by the Australian Learning and Teaching Council Ltd to develop the Assessment of Physiotherapy Practice (APP) instrument for assessment of physiotherapy students' clinical competency.

Dr Rod Fawns has had a significant presence in science education in Melbourne, Victoria for over 35 years, inspiring generations of science teachers as a leader in DipEd and MEd programs. He has been instrumental in developing many innovative teacher pre-service programs with a clear focus on the beginning teacher. Rod has been strongly involved with the Australian Science Teachers' Association and the Science Teachers' Association of Victoria (STAV). His contribution has been acknowledged with life membership of STAV. Rod has supervised and inspired a very large number of MEd and PhD students. He has been a long-time contributor and highly valued active member of the Australasian Science Education Research Association, and a prolific author of science education articles in areas of practical teaching and social theory. Rod also has a strong commitment to social and environmental issues.

Associate Professor Lynn Gillam is a bioethicist with particular interests in clinical ethics, genetics, research ethics and ethics education. She holds positions at three related institutions: The University of Melbourne, the Murdoch Children's Research Institute and the Royal Children's Hospital. Lynn currently teaches ethics in undergraduate and postgraduate programs, and supervises masters and PhD students. Lynn has 15 years' experience on Human Research Ethics Committees. She has published widely in bioethics, and is co-author of a text on critical thinking, *Facts and Values,* and *Telling Moments,* a narrative approach to clinical ethics. Her current research interests include pre-natal diagnosis and selective abortion; ethical decision making and the role of trust in research ethic; end-of-life decision making in paediatrics; and controversial medical treatments which alter children, in particular surgical treatment of intersex conditions. Lynn also has a strong interest in the intersections between ethics and sociology, and the development of interdisciplinary qualitative methods suitable for research in ethics.

Professor Rom Harré was for many years Lecturer in the Philosophy of Science at the University of Oxford. More recently he has been Distinguished Research Professor at Georgetown University in Washington DC. Currently he combines this with the Directorship of the Centre for the Philosophy of the Natural and Social Sciences at the London School of Economics. Rom has written widely on such topics as scientific realism and the foundations of physics. His recent books have been concerned with new directions in Social Psychology, particularly *Positioning Theory* with L van Langenhove.

Professor Joy Higgs is the Strategic Research Professor in Professional Practice and the Director of the Education for Practice Institute at Charles Sturt University, New South Wales. Previously Joy worked at The University of Sydney and The University of New South Wales. Her primary role is the advancement of practice-based education through collaborations in research, scholarship, student supervision and education. Joy has worked in health sciences education for over 26 years, and received a Member of the Order of Australia award for her contributions. Joy has produced over 300 publications including 14 books in her fields of expertise in professional practice, practice knowledge, clinical reasoning, qualitative research and professional education. In 2008 she published the third edition of *Clinical Reasoning in the Health Professions* with Mark Jones and colleagues. Joy is an experienced research supervisor, and in 2008 received an Australian Learning and Teaching Council Citation in recognition of her contributions to postgraduate research training.

Professor Jenny Keating is a physiotherapist with a PhD in musculoskeletal physiotherapy. She was appointed inaugural Professor and Head of Department of Physiotherapy at Monash University in 2005. Jenny has been the Course Convenor of the Bachelor of Physiotherapy programs and been actively writing and delivering the innovative new curricula with a committment to best practice in education. She is an active Cochrane reviewer and teaches research methods and statistical analysis to undergraduate physiotherapy students. The authors of Chapter 9 (Jenny Keating, Megan Dalton and Megan Davidson) have collaborated with physiotherapy educators Australia wide to develop a common method for assessing clinical competence of physiotherapy students.

Dr Sue Kilminster is Principal Research Fellow in the Medical Education Unit at the University of Leeds, the United Kingdom, and director of the Centre for Research into Professional Education. The rationale for establishing the centre was to explore and develop ways of integrating theoretical and empirical approaches to research in order to develop medical and healthcare professional education. Sue's current research interests include transitions, supervision and work-based learning, policy-related research, professionalism, assessment, interprofessional education and gender issues in medicine. Sue is a member of the course management team for the MEd in clinical education, and so involved in teaching and supervising students. Sue has worked in different areas of vocational and professional education and research for over 20 years and was previously a nurse.

Dr Stephen Loftus spent several years in clinical practice in dentistry in a variety of settings, from rural community clinics to oral and maxillofacial surgery units. More recently he has worked in undergraduate and postgraduate medical education for universities in both Europe and Australia. Stephen developed a research interest in clinical reasoning and how it is learned, while working in the multidisciplinary Pain Management and Research Centre of The University of Sydney. This interest led into exploring ways of using interpretive approaches to research clinical reasoning. He has been particularly inspired by the work of scholars such as Vygotsky, Wittgenstein, Gadamer and Bakhtin. He is also a co-editor of the latest editions of popular texts about clinical reasoning and communication in the health sciences.

Rosalind McDougall is a PhD student at The University of Melbourne, jointly enrolled at the Centre for Health and Society and the Centre for Applied Philosophy and Public Ethics. She completed a BPhil at the University of Oxford in 2005, focusing on medical ethics. Rosalind's current research investigates the ethical challenges faced by medical interns and residents.

Dr Silvia Mamede is a Scientific Researcher at the Institute of Psychology, Erasmus University, Rotterdam, where she works in studies on clinical reasoning and clinical education of medical students and physicians, undertaken in collaboration with the Faculty of Medicine. Silvia is a medical doctor, and completed her PhD on reflective practice in medicine at Erasmus University. Silvia previously worked in health professions' education for several years at the School of Public Health in Ceará, Brazil, and has continued to collaborate in the design and implementation of continuing education programs for family health physicians in Brazil. Her areas of research interest include clinical reasoning, reflective practice, clinical education, and continuing medical education.

Professor Henk Schmidt is the Dean of the Faculty of Social Sciences and Professor of Psychology at Erasmus University, Rotterdam, The Netherlands. His research areas of interest are learning and memory, in particular problem-based learning, long-term memory, and the development of expertise in medicine. Henk has published more than 250 articles in refereed journals, chapters in books, and books, alone or with more than 30 PhD students. In 2006 he received the Distinguished Career Award of the American Educational Research Association, Division I.

Robyn Smith is Health Services Manager, Allied Health Learning and Research at Northern Health, Victoria. Her role is to develop allied health staff capacity in research and evidence-based practice, and to foster excellence in clinical education and staff learning. She has led the development of a unique allied health interdisciplinary graduate program that supports the transition from student to professional, and the development and implementation of a supervision framework. Robyn is a lead contributor to Northern Health's development of a collaborative allied health clinical school. She was Chief Investigator on a recent project with La Trobe University, Faculty of Health Sciences, on Interprofessional Clinical Education for entry-level students. Prior to 2003, Robyn was Director of the Public Health Division at the National Ageing Research Institute (NARI), Melbourne. In almost 8 years at NARI she led a multidisciplinary research team completing more than 30 health services and clinical research projects in ageing, with the outcomes influencing policy and care for older people. Her clinical career included practice in acute aged care and adult rehabilitation. Robyn has completed an MPH, Grad Dip Gerontology and BAppSc (OT).

Nick Stone is currently a Senior Lecturer in Higher Education at the Centre for the Study of Higher Education, The University of Melbourne. He has worked across a wide range of education and training sectors and contexts, and managed the Rural Interprofessional Education (RIPE) Project from its inception to funding cessation 5 years later in 2006. Nick worked with Monash University as a Senior Lecturer in Interprofessional Education from 2006–07, and has provided a range of IP related consultancy services to other agencies. He has published in this and other areas. Nick also lectures Cross-cultural Management in the Department of Management at The University of Melbourne, and is completing a PhD titled 'Assessing Intercultural Effectiveness in Management Learning and Practice'. He sees strong connections between these areas and improving working relationships across and within the cultures of the health disciplines and professions.

Associate Professor Gillian Webb is the Director of Learning and Teaching at the School of Physiotherapy, The University of Melbourne. She has been in health professional education for more than three decades. Gillian has a masters in Clinical Education and a PhD in Education. Her research has focused on clinical education models, students' formation of their professional identity, as well as more general health educational issues. She is the Chairperson of the Educators Group of the Australian Physiotherapy Association and President of the International Society of Physiotherapy Educators. She has had extensive experience in curriculum planning and design in Australia and in countries in the Asia-Pacific region.

Dr Robyn Woodward-Kron is a Senior Lecturer in the Medical Education Unit at The University of Melbourne and coordinates the Faculty's International Student Support Program. She has a PhD in educational linguistics. Her teaching and research interests are language and learning, discourse analysis, and intercultural clinical communication. Robyn is one of the authors of the DVD-ROM *'I'm feeling a bit crook': Understanding and managing clinical communication in Australia*. Current projects include developing multimedia resources for international medical graduates on teaching effective and ethical clinical communication, and developing clinical communication feedback guidelines for international medical graduate workplace-based assessment.

Introduction

This book aims to advance knowledge construction and application in clinical education through presenting theories, models and empirical findings. Clinical settings are dynamic educational spaces that present both opportunities and barriers to learning and teaching. Changing patient populations, and changing practice knowledge driven by research and global changes in communication and information technology, add to the complexity of this learning environment. Institutional and organisational factors of the hospital, clinic or community placement and the university also impact on teaching and learning. Hierarchies of authority in clinical decision making, limited resources, and varying policy directives and agendas of workplaces all add to the complexity of the clinical education setting. This complexity challenges students and educators to learn to adapt their knowledge and practices, to meet diverse needs of patients and families, and to work effectively with other members of the healthcare team. This book highlights these layers of complexity in clinical education and encourages educators to recognise teaching and learning opportunities within this unique environment.

The models of practice that might be used to shed light on the clinical education environment and its particular features, challenges and opportunities, are based on explanatory theories. For example, theories of workplace learning, theories about learning within professional communities, theories about supervisor and student relationships, and theories that explain the influence of culture in learning, all provide perspectives and frameworks from which teaching and learning methods can be developed, tested and better understood.

This book seeks to encourage debate and dialogue from a broad range of clinical educators, and to highlight the inherent complexity of clinical education knowledge and practice. It encourages the reader to challenge their own educational practices that may be speculatively or historically based, rather than grounded in empirical research or theoretical principles. Each of the chapters presents insights into clinical education based on observations of practice, and from research quantitatively measuring or qualitatively exploring clinical education practices. The result is a composite of ideas and research on many facets of clinical education relevant to a range of health professional educators.

At the beginning of each chapter, we identify key theoretical frameworks and assumptions made by the author(s). We then suggest how these theories might be used to inform clinical education curriculum design or research. From this basis, teaching methods and examples are also proposed.

The book is divided into three sections that cover broad but distinctive features of learning and teaching in the clinical setting. The first concerns theories of professional knowledge including its construction by students and educators, and its application in clinical placement settings (critical reflection, ways of knowing and theory, research and practice in clinical education). The second section includes chapters that focus on the influence of contexts and communities on teaching and learning processes in clinical education (professional identities and communities of practice, interprofessional education, and embracing diversity). The third section integrates theories of knowledge construction with educational methods by focusing on discrete facets of clinical education curricula (clinical reasoning, feedback, assessment and ethics).

Learning clinical skills relies on acquiring a body of theoretical and fact-based knowledge that is discipline specific. It also requires practical or technique-based knowledge and skills applied to a range of clinical scenarios and patient circumstances. Methods for teaching effective acquisition and application of knowledge required for clinical practice has been, and continues to be, the focus of sustained research and theory development. These theoretical perspectives are discussed in Section 1 'Examining knowledge: theoretical perspectives about knowledge construction'.

In Chapter 1 'Critical reflection in clinical education: beyond the "swampy lowlands"', Clare Delany and Elizabeth Molloy discuss theories that provide a framework for thinking critically and reflectively in clinical practice. Throughout their commentary they illustrate the central theme of the book, the importance of identification and, in turn, integration of theory, evidence and practice in clinical education. The authors present what they have termed the 'iterative model of critical reflection', in which critical reflection is described as an active, spiraling and open-ended skill that facilitates increased understanding of and capacity to critique and change established practice knowledge. Through this model, they suggest that for students to incorporate habits of critical reflection in their professional practice, methods of teaching and assessment of such skills must include explicit links with underlying explanatory theories, and should be modelled and integrated within all aspects of the curriculum.

Two examples of how the iterative model of critical reflection might be used in clinical education curricula are presented. The first is an overview of a range of different tasks vertically integrated over a four-year physiotherapy curriculum. The second is an extended excerpt from a student's reflective writing as an example of the potential learning value in reflective writing. The authors argue that drawing on underpinning explanatory theories, vertically integrating reflection activities into curricula design, and encouraging educators to model reflective practice, all work to position critical reflection as a relevant and important part of professional practice, rather than a peripheral and extra-curricular task imposed on students by educators.

In Chapter 2 'Ways of knowing for clinical practice', Joy Higgs presents theoretical perspectives underpinning the nature of professional knowledge and how it is constructed by educators and students. The focus is on how health practice knowledge has evolved, including its dependence upon sociocultural and historical understandings of professional practice. Higgs provides an overview of the models of healthcare practice and their associated learning and teaching strategies, ranging from the apprenticeship model to the interactional person-centred professional. The historical and sociocultural influences on the development of professional knowledge and practice are then identified. Higgs suggests that ways of knowing and practising need to be understood within the current sociocultural context, including community expectations of practice. The implications for clinical education are that teaching needs to be clearly linked to the nature and development of clinical practice knowledge, so that clinical educators and students are empowered to interact from an informed, sensitive and reflexive basis within the current clinical practice environment.

In the third chapter 'Recognising and bridging gaps: theory, research and practice in clinical education', Sue Kilminster provides further discussion about the nature and theoretical bases of teaching and learning in clinical education. She discusses two theoretical perspectives that are relevant to underpin learning in clinical education. They are cognitive psychology (a theoretical perspective that focuses on how knowledge is internally constructed and acquired by individual learners) and the sociocultural paradigm (emphasising learning as constructing knowledge through participation).

Kilminster contends that the assumptions underpinning learning in the clinical context need to be made explicit to facilitate, develop and advance relevant clinical education pedagogy. She proposes a research paradigm of workplace learning and teaching as a possible way to develop more integrated approaches to frame and link research, clinical practice and clinical education. The elements in this paradigm include movement from peripheral to full participation; access to goals for performance; direct guidance of experts and others; and indirect guidance provided by the workplace. In presenting these elements, Kilminster sets the scene for examining learning and teaching as contextually and socially bound activites.

The key message Kilminster presents is that if learning, and research about learning, is understood from a sociocultural perspective in combination with the cognitive view of knowledge acquisition, then the divide between clinical practice and clinical education can be reformulated.

The first three chapters challenge the reader to go beyond describing 'what seems to work' and how learning outcomes might be measured in the clinical context. Instead educators are asked to examine the nature of clinical knowledge and the mechanisms that may enhance or constrain learning in the clinical environment. In the area of critical reflection, the reader is encouraged to not only promote critical reflection as a learning activity for students, but to understand the theoretical bases of reflection and to model these in their own practices. When considering the aims of clinical education more generally, the reader is encouraged to reframe their thinking about practice and associated research. In Chapter 3, Kilminster poses the following questions to trigger re-conceptualisation, and such questions can be applied to processes and practices critiqued throughout the book:

- What is the nature of clinical knowledge?
- How does an individual come to possess it?
- How can they be helped in the process?
- How can we all know that a professional does 'possess' the requisite knowledge?

Section 2 'Sharing knowledge: communities and culture in education' moves from a focus on critical thinking and knowledge construction to the nature and influence of communities and culture on clinical education practices. In Chapter 4 'Professional identities and communities of practice', Gillian Webb, Rod Fawns and Rom Harré present two theoretical frameworks that provide different perspectives and ways of understanding communication, relationships and discourse in the clinical education environments. They refer to Vygosky's (1962) theory on psychological symbiosis to explain the interconnected nature of cognition and identity, and how conversations can shape professional identity in the clinical setting. Through this theory, the authors argue that institutional socialisation is a dynamic process where students, bringing their own 'story-lines', and through their articulation, can influence the community of practice. Examples are provided to illustrate the learner's professional socialisation, and the mutual responsibility of learner and teacher in generating learning opportunities and sharing story-lines in the clinical context.

The second theoretical perspective presented in this chapter is derived from aspects of Vygotsky's work. Harré's 'Positioning Theory' is presented as a tool that practitioners and students might use to facilitate reflection and examination of their clinical and educational interactions. The key contention is that the lens of Positioning Theory enables greater critique of the metaphorical 'positions' adopted by educators and learners, and how these relational activities impact on learning. Both theories have applicability in research and practice in clinical education, where learning and instruction occur in practice communities and through professional discourse.

In Chapter 5, Megan Davidson, Robyn Smith and Nick Stone move from the previous chapters' discussion of theoretical concepts that underpin learning within a discipline-specific community to a focus on how professional communities might practise at an interdisciplinary level. Their title 'Interprofessional education: sharing the wealth' suggests that interprofessional education (IPE) presents an opportunity for collaborative work that has advantages for all participants. The authors contend that in addition to reflecting the tenets of a patient-centred approach to health care, interprofessional practice (IPP) has the potential for many practical benefits in areas of knowledge generation, healthcare outcomes and, more globally, from a healthcare economics perspective. The chapter describes specific advantages of interprofessional education and practice and provides examples of evidence of the benefits of IPE and IPP. The perceived barriers to implementing IPE are identified with some suggested responses to these challenges. The authors draw from their own experience in curriculum design, and from research that has evaluated the effects of IPE.

In Chapter 6 'Clinical education: embracing diversity', Anna Chur-Hansen and Robyn Woodward-Kron highlight the variation and cultural diversity in health professional practice communities, and suggest how this diversity might be used as a resource in clinical education. The authors identify literature that discusses the challenges of diversity for clinical educators, students and health professionals. Such challenges include language expertise (including the use of informal and colloquial language), and varying experiences in the biopsychosocial and biomedical approaches to the treatment encounter. Within this literature, the authors highlight an ongoing debate about the use of traditional models of biomedical practice to understand cultural competency. The authors suggest that presenting culture as static, homogeneous and linked with ethnicity fails to recognise that biomedicine is a culture in itself. They draw on constructs from medical anthropology and linguistics to present models of approaching teaching and learning within diverse cultural environments. Concepts of 'cultural competence,' models of health and illness, and analytic frameworks using linguistics are explored to inform clinical practice and education.

From a practical perspective, the authors argue that teaching cultural competence needs to be integrated into the core curriculum rather than positioned as a 'once-off' workshop or lecture. In addition, they recommend that simulated patients, standardised patient encounters, role-plays, reflective journals and feedback from educators and patients are key educational methods to develop skills in cultural competence. Although the authors state that evaluation of cultural competency training interventions is key to improving curricula design and implementation, they also highlight the potential problems with assessing 'facts' about culture that may inadvertently lead to the encouragement of stereotyping.

The four chapters in the final section 'Applying knowledge: teaching and learning practices' all focus on ways to integrate theories, evidence and knowledge of clinical education by identifying specific areas of the clinical education curriculum. Each of these chapters aims to increase educators' understanding about their role in implementing aspects of the curriculum through acknowledging students' perspectives, facilitating student agency and increasing the understanding of theories that underpin components of clinical education. The curricular areas described are clinical reasoning, feedback, assessment, and ethics.

In Chapter 7 'Clinical reasoning: the nuts and bolts of clinical education', Rola Ajjawi, Stephen Loftus; Henk Schmidt and Silvia Mamede provide two alternative but complementary models to understand and examine the clinical reasoning process. In the first half of the chapter the authors draw on models of reasoning founded in behaviourism and cognitivism, and highlight key features of 'the stage theory' of knowledge acquisition and development of expertise in health professions. In the second half they refer to the interpretivist paradigm 'as a complementary way to understand' the process of teaching and learning clinical reasoning. The authors contend that the interpretivist paradigm resonates with the way that experienced practitioners develop their reasoning capability within a professional community of practice.

The models presented in this chapter suggest that combining or at least being aware of the theoretical frameworks that underpin the clinical reasoning process expands the range of teaching possibilities. Educators are encouraged to not only direct students' attention to salient cognitive and contextual features in clinical learning situations, but also to encourage novices to engage with their practice community and to talk about their practice with others. In this chapter, one model is not privileged over another. Instead, the authors propose that by understanding frameworks about clinical reasoning, educators can choose between them to fit particular teaching and learning purposes. The chapter encourages the reader to ask and find answers to questions that were similarly posed in Chapter 1 about clinical education in general. That is:

- What is clinical reasoning?
- What are the epistemological underpinnings of the prevalent models of clinical reasoning taught in health professional curricula?
- How is clinical reasoning best taught in the clinical context?

In Chapter 8 'Time to pause: giving and receiving feedback in clinical education', Elizabeth Molloy presents a synthesis of ideas on best practice feedback based on a review of the literature. In addition, key findings from her empirical research examining feedback in clinical education are highlighted. Molloy identifies that educators' descriptions of effective feedback practice were congruent with the espoused principles of 'best practice feedback' in the literature. However, despite both educators' and students' acknowledgement of the importance of two-way feedback interactions, their enactment of feedback in the clinical education setting was distinctly different to their self-reports of practice. Molloy's research demonstrates that both students and educators are complicit in enacting an educator-driven, one-way feedback culture. Some of the factors contributing to this disjunction between theory and practice include lack of time, lack of knowledge on feedback philosophy, adherence by educators to a clinical 'diagnostic script', and issues of power within the supervisor–student relationship.

Recommendations for understanding and implementing effective feedback in clinical education are provided with the aim of developing increased agency and capacity for self-evaluation in the recipient of the feedback. Molloy's empirically based strategies for improving educators' ability to give feedback encourage a shift in feedback practices away from 'diagnostic and prescriptive' information provision towards that of a two-way conversation. Reflecting the importance of enhancing agency, this chapter highlights 'feedback' conversations in clinical education as a vehicle for students to develop shared meanings and contribute to the discourse of the profession.

In Chapter 9 'Assessment in clinical education', Jenny Keating, Megan Dalton and Megan Davidson argue for the importance and relevance of formative assessment in clinical education. That is, the ability to monitor students over a sufficiently long period of time to enable observation of practice in a range of circumstances and across a spectrum of patient types and needs. They also highlight a number of challenges educators might encounter that may act to decrease the validity, reliability and fairness of the assessment process in clinical education. These include educator bias, potential confusion between assessing outcomes rather than methods of treatments, and over reliance on summative assessment.

On the basis of these contentions, the authors provide a detailed description of the development, testing and implementation of a performance-based assessment tool in physiotherapy contexts, Assessment of Physiotherapy Practice (APP). Through careful explication of their research methodology, the authors suggest this assessment tool might address many of the inherent challenges of assessment in clinical education. In particular, they highlight that the unique and most useful aspects of the clinical assessment tool is its clear criteria, which can be linked to explicit performance indicators. They contend that explicit performance indicators work to reduce assessor bias, in addition to providing students with clear practice goals. As items on the APP are drawn from generic competencies expected of all healthcare providers, the authors suggest the tool and its method of development is applicable to other health practice disciplines.

In the final chapter 'Ethics in clinical education', Clare Delany, Lynn Gillam and Rosalind McDougall use ethics education to draw together two of the key messages of the book—the importance of being aware of the sources of knowledge in clinical education curricula, and the potential effects of different ways of teaching that knowledge. The authors acknowledge the centrality of ethics education to health professional practice. They discuss trends that can be seen across the different health professions, or 'strands' representing different aspects or parts of the whole picture of ethics education. The five strands identified by the authors include ethics as decision making, character and attitude, advocacy, moral agency, and ethics as professional identity.

The authors suggest that an awareness of the origin and development of the different strands, including how and why different health professions have incorporated them into their ethics education, provides many potential advantages for ethics curricula developers. Within these strands, the authors reason there are potential ideas and resources to combat the threats to ethical practice and to address gaps between what is taught as theoretical ideas of ethical practice and the realities of clinical practice.

Examining how the strands relate to the ethical issues encountered in clinical practice is an important way to develop relevant and effective ethics curricula.

Section 1

Examining knowledge: theoretical perspectives about knowledge construction

CHAPTER 1

Critical reflection in clinical education: beyond the 'swampy lowlands'

Clare Delany and Elizabeth Molloy

THEORIES

Three theories that underpin critical reflection are introduced in this chapter. *Reflexivity* is a theoretical framework that recognises the influence of one's own perspective and methods of constructing knowledge. *Postmodernist* ideas represent theoretical perspectives that argue for complexity and competing understandings of knowledge construction. *Critical theory* highlights the influence of the social world, including hierarchies of knowledge and power in the development of knowledge and practice.

USING THEORIES TO INFORM CURRICULUM DESIGN AND RESEARCH

When designing health practice curricula that incorporate critical reflection, each of these theories may be used to frame ways to reflect on learning experiences and research. Using reflexivity means the curriculum should provide an opportunity for students to understand how their personal and discipline-specific perspectives impact on their learning or their interaction with others. Using postmodernist perspectives means critical reflection learning tasks should be designed to encourage students to explore and experience alternative views to those of their own health professional discipline. As an underlying theoretical framework, critical theory means the curriculum or research about the curriculum should enhance students' acknowledgement and understanding of historical and sociocultural views of their own practice and learning experiences within the broader healthcare system.

3

USING THEORIES TO DRIVE EDUCATION METHODS

Critical reflection learning tasks should incorporate opportunities for students to enquire into the theories of knowledge construction that underpin thinking, writing and speaking, critically and reflectively. Methods of teaching students could include not only providing them with an opportunity to describe and analyse an event, but also opportunities to express how their description and analysis relates to other perspectives, theories and understandings of that event. In this way, teaching students how to critically reflect teaches them how to not only recognise the swampy lowlands of clinical practice but also to move freely within or beyond them.

Introduction

In healthcare practice, thinking reflectively means thinking about and evaluating experiences in order to reach new understandings and perspectives (Schön 1983, 1987, Boud et al 1985). Thinking critically means unearthing deeper assumptions or pre-suppositions about practice (Mezirow 1991, Fook 2004), about power (Brookfield 1995), and about connections between oneself and social contexts (Fook 2004). When these two meanings are combined, 'critical reflection' involves a process of both change and challenge to professional practice. Critical reflection, described in this way, also implies that the teaching of critical reflection skills should not be confined to a discrete 'package' in health professional education, but rather positioned as relevant and integral to thinking in all aspects of health professional curricula.

In this chapter, we describe a theoretical model of critical reflection that we label the 'iterative model of critical reflection'. As the label suggests, we see critical reflection as an active and open-ended skill that uses the process of thinking about practice to better understand, challenge and critique established practice knowledge. Through our model, we argue that for students to develop habits of critical reflection in their professional practice, methods of teaching and assessing such skills must incorporate explicit links with underlying explanatory theories, and must be modelled and integrated within all aspects of the curriculum.

To illustrate how the iterative model of critical reflection might be implemented in clinical education, we present an example of vertical integration of a critical reflection program within an undergraduate physiotherapy curriculum. We also include an extended example and analysis of one student's reflective writing essay from this undergraduate program. In presenting our iterative model of critical reflection and the way it informs curriculum content, we hope to increase awareness and promote a deeper understanding of how skills in critical reflection might be more meaningfully incorporated into health professional education.

Critical reflection, healthcare practice and education

The healthcare context is recognised as an uncertain (Higgs & Titchen 2001), continuously changing (Ryan et al 2003), 'swampy' or messy (Schön 1987) working environment. The qualities that health practitioners require to practise in such an environment include being autonomous, confident, self-directed, ethical, flexible, collaborative, inclusive, organised and innovative (Ryan et al 2003). Iedema et al (2004) categorise these personal qualities into three types of abilities. The first is a level of reflexivity about the paradigms of knowledge that underpin specific healthcare practices. The second, an ability to understand and work with other health practitioners, and the third, an ability to articulate complex descriptions of different knowledge domains contributing to health practices.

Higgs and Titchen (2001) similarly outline teaching, learning and practice strategies that are necessary to promote these abilities and to reframe the interface between an uncertain world of professional practice and health professional education. They include:

1 developing a greater (and more critical) understanding of professional knowledge
2 being attentive to personal and professional values, and understanding underpinning healthcare practice
3 generating theories of knowledge derived from practical experience
4 incorporating practice knowledge into educational curricula so that students receive preparation for professional work from both propositional (factual) and emerging practice knowledge (experiential).

In recognition of both the clinical practice environment, and the required qualities and abilities that practitioners need to continue to develop as professionals, methods of promoting and teaching skills in critical reflection have received increasing attention in clinical education literature (Higgs & Titchen 2001, Dye 2005, Jensen et al 1990, Maudsley & Strivens 2000, Henderson & Johnson 2002, Trede et al 2003, Cole et al 2004). Teaching skills of critical reflection in health education has been proposed as a means to counter a positivist tendency in health sciences education to present knowledge and clinical skills in terms of measurable mastery and attainment of specific competencies (Kneebone 2002). Thinking critically and reflectively has been identified as one way to counter teaching strategies that rely on uncritical knowledge transfer between teachers and students. This knowledge transfer approach is a feature of experiential learning through an apprenticeship model, where students are exposed to a range of clinical scenarios and conditions through observation initially, and then through supervised clinical practice (McLeod et al 1997, Dornan et al 2007). In this model, there is an emphasis on the learner 'acquiring knowledge and skills from an expert or master with the goal of emulating their expertise' (Higgs & Titchen 2001).

Recent critiques of experiential learning and use of apprenticeship models suggest that they focus on building individually based, discipline-specific knowledge, operational competence and outcomes (Rees 2004, Bleakley 2006), and neglect the idea that professional learning and practice involves adaptive, sociocultural and heuristic or interpretive processes (Eraut 1994, Jensen et al 2000, Edwards et al 2004, Talbot 2004, Bleakley 2006). On the basis of these critiques, experiential learning may not be enough to meet the need for health professionals to be flexible, aware and have an understanding of alternative perspectives held by patients, healthcare professionals, hospital administrators and others (Trede et al 2003).

Critical reflection skills are recognised as a response to these critiques because they represent a way of thinking for students and practitioners to analyse the domains of knowledge underpinning their practice and to enable them to learn from, and redevelop, their practice (Kember 2001, Fook 2004). This role has also been reinforced by studies that demonstrate a link between the skills and use of critical reflection and the development of expertise in healthcare practice (Shepard et al 1999, Edwards et al 2004, Dye 2005, Jensen et al 2000).

Critical reflection is therefore seen to have a role in both enhancing the learning process itself and as a means of professional development (Pee et al 2002).

Models of critical reflection

The original proponents of reflection in professional practice refer to a series of steps to follow and an underlying rationale to guide the reflective process. Dewey (1933) described separate phases of problem definition, problem analysis, formulation of a theory of action and then action. The key characteristic of this process is one of careful consideration of actions by delaying initial reactions and developing an understanding of alternative options and perspectives.

Schön (1987) distinguished between different types of reflection by describing the process of reflecting-on-action and reflecting-in-action. The latter category requires practitioners to maintain a sense of curiosity and openness while they practise, to enable them to recognise and challenge their own implicit understanding and interpretation of a clinical situation. Schön's two types of reflection have been incorporated into various models of reflective practice, designed to provide a structure and process for students to follow.

Baird and Winter (2005) describe three models of reflection to guide teaching and learning strategies that facilitate reflective thinking and practice. The first of these was originally proposed by Boud (1993). In this model, students are encouraged to first identify their personal experiences that act to inform their learning intentions. Second, to describe the clinical learning or practice experience by explicitly building on their own understanding and knowledge. The third and final step involves a re-examination and evaluation of their learning experiences.

The Gibbs (1988) circular model follows six phases. The first two are descriptive. Students are required to describe the learning or clinical event, including their accompanying feelings. This is followed by a two-step evaluative phase, where the value and meaning of the experience is questioned and discussed. The final two steps involve thinking about and articulating alternative actions and planning for future actions in light of the lessons learnt.

Another commonly applied model proposed by Driscoll (2000) is a series of steps. The steps include description, analysis and evaluation. They are similar to the model proposed by Gibbs, with the addition of a seventh step to encourage the student to plan how to put into action the new learning gained from reflecting on the clinical practice experience.

Methods of 'doing' critical reflection

Critical reflection has received considerable attention in a range of health professions, including nursing (Howell 1989, Johns 1995), social work (Taylor & White 2000, Gardner 2003, Fook 2004), medicine (Maudsley & Strivens 2000, Henderson & Johnson 2002, Cole et al 2004, Iedema et al 2004), dentistry (Pee et al 2002), occupational therapy (Routledge et al 1997) and physiotherapy (Cross 1993, Larin et al 2005). This body of literature describes two main methods to incorporate reflection into health education curricula.

The most common is via reflective diaries or journals (Larin et al 2005, Dye 2005, Francis 1995, Richardson & Maltby 1995, Routledge et al 1997, Snadden & Thomas 1998, Chirema 2007, Clouder 2000, Cross 1997). One rationale underlying this method is that by setting a structured task of journal writing, students will establish a habit of reflection and be encouraged to develop ongoing skills in critical reflection.

Another common method for encouraging student reflection is through structured verbal feedback sessions between student and educator (Ende et al 1995, Frye et al 1997, Molloy & Clarke 2005). These feedback opportunities are generally integrated into the clinical education curriculum. In these situations, the clinical educator provides feedback about how the student is progressing, and the student is expected to reflect either verbally or via a written self-assessment form about their own learning progress. Within these feedback sessions, clinical educators are expected to facilitate students' reflective capacity through the skilled use of questions and prompts (see Ch 8). The collaborative generation of insights represents a form of critical reflection of the student's performance, and is used to guide strategies for improvement, and the setting of new learning goals (Henderson et al 2005).

Studies that describe methods of introducing critical reflection within health professional curricula as either written or verbal tasks, have assessed the outcome and effectiveness of students' critical reflection on the basis of how critical or analytical the writing is and by how students' reflections change over time. In the latter category, longitudinally based studies have identified that as students progress through their clinical training, the *content* of their reflective writing changes from a focus on themselves as learners (Jensen et al 2000, Cross 1993) to a focus and increased insight into the importance of understanding the patient's perspective (Wessel & Larin 2006). Studies that discuss the outcome of students' reflective writing in terms of how it demonstrates levels of critique and analysis, focus on the *process* of reflection (Boenink et al 2004, Pee et al 2002, Henderson & Johnson 2002). Assessment of critical reflection tasks from this 'process perspective' measure student reflection on the basis of whether it is (Hatton & Smith 1995):

- descriptive and merely reports events without providing reasons;
- reflectively descriptive, providing reasons based on personal judgements, without evaluation of the personal judgement;
- reflective through dialogue, where reasons and alternatives are posed but not necessarily answered within the reflective process; or
- critically reflective, where consideration is given to the socio-political context, including roles, relationships, gender, professional views and knowledge, that might shape events and decisions.

A further debate about assessment of critical reflection concerns whether or not students' reflective capacity should be assessed at all (Rose & Best 2005, Cross 1993). The claim against assessment of reflective practice is generally based on the premise that external assessment may constrain honest reflections by students. As a counter to this claim, we suggest that assessment of critical reflection writing provides students with structure for their reflection, feedback on the depth of their reflective capacity, and, most importantly, reinforcement of the integral role that reflection plays in healthcare education and practice. However, students need to be reassured that their reflective writing is not assessed according to the stance or viewpoints they take, but rather their degree of engagement in the process of critical reflection (Driessen et al 2005).

The shared feature of each of these models, and the assessment and teaching methods they support, is an emphasis on the process of reflection and the explicit steps to follow. These steps are important to describe clearly because they provide a framework to guide different methods of critical reflection. However, we contend that unless the different critical reflection tasks are absorbed into the fabric of professional ways of learning, teaching and practising, their ability to be practically useful and to lead to sustainable habits of professional practice is limited. Some of the factors that may act to limit the absorption or integration of critical reflection into the fabric of health professional practice and curricula include:

- a lack of conceptual underpinning of critical reflection tasks
- a focus on *description* and *analysis* of incidents and practice rather than a prompt to use the reflection to *change* and *challenge* practice
- a lack of vertical integration of reflective tasks in the academic program to enable incremental building of critical reflection skills
- a lack of modelling of critical reflection by both academic and clinical staff.

These factors may act as potential barriers to the integration of critical reflection. They are addressed in the iterative critical reflection model, discussed below.

The iterative model of critical reflection

In developing our 'iterative model of critical reflection', we aimed to embed the tenets of critical reflection within and across the curriculum. This involved more than setting a series of tasks that facilitated critical reflection. It involved teaching the theories that underpin the steps of critical reflection and promoting the use of these theories as a means for students to individually and personally interpret, apply and develop new knowledge when engaging in new tasks. Using this model, the learning process becomes an iterative one that relies on students going back to underpinning theories to inform their critical reflection tasks in much the same way that they rely on theories of practice to inform their clinical discipline-based knowledge (Fig 1.1).

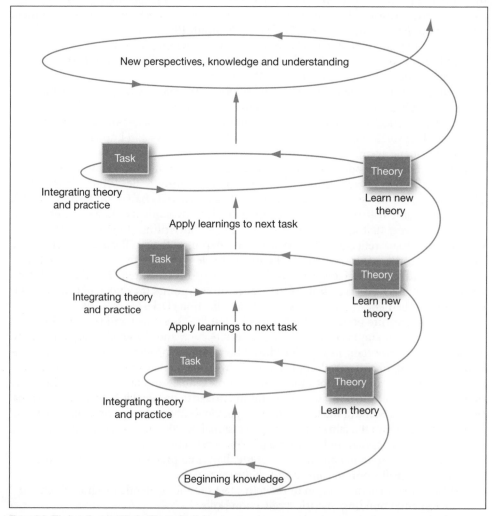

Figure 1.1 The iterative model of critical reflection

Our iterative model draws from the work of Fook (2002, 2004) who developed a model of critical reflection in social work practice. Fook (2004) linked ideas of reflective practice with underlying theoretical bases of reflexivity, postmodernism and critical theory. These theoretical perspectives and intellectual traditions provide important underlying explanations for the critical reflection program described in this chapter.

The process of using theoretical principles to inform practice is well established in the science and evidence underpinning healthcare practice (Kneebone 2002, Herbert et al 2005). For example, there is a clear expectation that in order for students to describe the steps involved in assessing an ankle sprain, they need to have an underlying knowledge of theories of the inflammatory cascade, the healing process, and the effect of load on collagen deposition. In the same way, we believe critical reflection tasks that require students to construct, interpret, evaluate and reflect on experiential knowledge, including a range of perspectives, must also be explicated in terms of underlying theories. We contend that this familiarity with, and acceptance of, the theoretical knowledge base that underpins reflective practice, mean that students will more likely develop habits of reflection as an integral component of their professional practice. The model presented in this chapter has been applied and evaluated in a specific critical reflection program for undergraduate physiotherapy students (Delany & Watkin 2008). Student and facilitator evaluation of the program highlighted themes of validation and sharing; a break in clinical performance and a broadening of their spheres of knowledge. These themes resonated with students' overall experiences of learning in clinical placements, and the research provides some evidence for the inclusion of critical reflection as a valid and worthwhile component of early clinical education.

Theories underpinning critical reflection
Theory one: reflexivity

The idea of reflexivity has traditionally been associated with paradigms of qualitative research (Barry et al 1999, Patton 2002, Hansen 2006) but is increasingly recognised as important in healthcare practice (Taylor & White 2000, Jensen 2005). Guillemin and Gillam (2004, p 269) describe reflexivity in qualitative research as a process involving critical reflection of how the researcher constructs knowledge from the research process. According to Patton (2002, p 65), it reminds the researcher to be attentive to and conscious of 'the cultural, political, social, linguistic and ideological origins' of first, their own perspective and voice; second, the perspectives and voices of those they interview; and third, the perspectives of those to whom the research is reported. Reflexivity has clear links with reflective practice because it seeks to increase awareness of how personal values and beliefs interconnect with other perspectives and with social and environmental contexts (Boud et al 1985). Patton (2002, p 66) suggests a number of reflexive questions as a framework to guide 'reflexive interrogation' in qualitative research. We have re-labelled (in italics) these questions because they represent questions that are relevant to how reflexivity as a qualitative research construct connects with critical reflection in clinical practice.

1 Researcher/*student*/*practitioner* perspective
- What do I know?
- How do I know what I know?
- What shapes and has shaped my perspective?
- With what voice do I share my perspective?
- What do I do with what I have found?

2 Participants'/*patients'* perspective
   - How do they know what they know?
   - What shapes and has shaped their world view?
   - How do they perceive me and why?
   - How do I perceive them?
3 Audience/*colleagues'*/*supervisors'* perspective
   - How do they make sense of what I give them?
   - What perspectives do they bring to the findings I offer?
   - How do they perceive me?

The notion of reflexivity applied to clinical practice encompasses an awareness of the different roles and perspectives that practitioners, students, patients and educators bring to their treatment encounters. Reflexivity is based on the theoretical assumption that people do not share one perspective or one version of reality. This theoretical view of knowledge and practice enables analysis of personal learning experiences to move from a *description* to a *critique* of influences, knowledge and perspectives. Recognising and taking seriously alternative perspectives and ways of knowing and understanding is sometimes more broadly labelled as postmodernism. This framework of knowledge forms the second theoretical premise of the iterative critical reflection model.

Theory two: postmodernism

Postmodernist theories argue for descriptions of knowledge and versions of reality that recognise the world as 'complex, overlaid with competing and perhaps contradictory understandings' (Rice & Ezzy 1999, p 21). Fook (2004) interprets postmodernist theory as a challenge to modernist (linear, unified and positivist) thinking in clinical practice contexts. Fook's practical interpretation of postmodernism is to encourage students to value and expect uncertainty, and to be modest or at least self aware in relation to their own position within multiple realities and perspectives (Pease & Fook 1999). Understood in this way, postmodernism provides a framework to construct and deconstruct meaning and knowledge through conversation and dialogue. It provides a theoretical standpoint to break down barriers created by privileged positions and knowledge.

Schön (1987) also highlighted the value of the postmodernist perspective in his description of the 'swampy lowland' of everyday practice. Schön's argument for reflective practice derived from his challenge to the positivist epistemology that underpinned university education. He argued that such a framework emphasising 'technical rationality' misrepresented how professionals think and act.

> In the varied topography of professional practice, there is a high, hard ground where practitioners can make effective use of research-based theory and technique, and there is a swampy lowland where situations are confusing 'messes' incapable of technical solution. (Schön 1983, p 42)

One criticism of postmodernism, especially as it applies to professional knowledge and practice, is that while it enables critique and analysis of unified and hegemonic systems of knowledge and practice, it does not provide a way of definitively acting in clinical practice. Pease and Fook (1999) explicitly adopt a stance of 'weak postmodernism', which they define as one that values empiricism and unified knowledge but positions such knowledge as one of the many perspectives of professional work. This theoretical framework provides a pathway to include and notice the influence of social, cultural and emotional perspectives on the process of learning and practising, while recognising the integral nature of being informed by empirically based theories of knowledge and practice.

Implicit in both reflexivity and postmodernism is an acknowledgement of the importance of recognising and being informed by other perspectives, personal experiences and different ways of understanding practice. Although the models of critical reflection described earlier are premised on these underlying theories, labelling the steps as being derived from theories of postmodernism, reflexivity and, as discussed below, critical theory, provides more explicit frameworks from which students and practitioners can describe, interpret and understand their learning and practice experiences.

Theory three: critical theory

Critical theory focuses on the influence of the social world, including hierarchies of knowledge and power in the development of knowledge and practice (Higgs & Titchen 2001). Being 'critical', in this theoretical sense, means being mindful of the factors that culturally and historically influence clinical learning and experience. Critical theory, in the context of clinical practice and learning, is an important underlying theory because it provides a way to describe and distinguish between empirically established and historically based 'reality' and the personal 'reality' of students, patients, clinical educators and other members of the healthcare team. Importantly, a critical view of reflecting on how practice knowledge is generated has the potential to transform a student's knowledge from acceptance of established ways of knowing that do not challenge or seek to understand the influence of hierarchies of authority, to a richer and more nuanced understanding of the influences and factors involved. Critical theory can therefore act as a transformatory or emancipatory theory of learning and practising (Trede et al 2003). Transformative learning is an area of educational theory and practice (Mezirow 1991) that encourages learning through critical self reflection of assumptions, beliefs, practices and ways of seeing the world. Use of critical theory to inform critical reflection means empowering students to understand the influence of habitual views and ways of understanding people, contexts and practices, and to develop an openness to different frames of reference.

Iterative critical reflection

The final component of our model of iterative critical reflection, and the point that distinguishes it from Fook's model of critical reflection, is our emphasis on the iterative character of critical reflection built into the health professional curriculum. In qualitative research, the term 'iterative' is used to describe the conscious movement between data and relevant theory to build understanding (Hansen 2006). It is a process of analysing and critically reflecting on the meaning of the data in relation to theories that help to explain or provide an account for the data. When applied to critical reflection in clinical practice, iterative reflection means moving between a description of an event and a search for an explanatory framework that helps to support an interpretation, or provide increased insight into a learning or practice event. From this new understanding built from both personal and theoretical knowledge bases, we contend it is possible to gain insight into practice and to identify alternative responses for the future.

Use of the term 'iterative' helps to distinguish our model from previously described models of reflection. We aim to encourage students to explicitly refer to theories of knowledge that underpin their interpretation or understanding of their experience. In the reflective step that requires students to make sense of or interpret their clinical experience, we suggest that students should choose from propositional knowledge (empirically based); personal experience that includes their own way of understanding knowledge (reflexivity); theories that relate to student–supervisor relationships or other historical ways of understanding how people position themselves as learners, teachers, patients and managers (critical theory); and theories that might offer ways to understand different perspectives of people and institutional systems (postmodernism). We contend that this iterative movement between theories of knowledge and practice experience provides a stable theoretical platform upon which methods of critical reflection can be based.

Moving iteratively between different theories of knowledge and understanding also provides a way for educators to engage with and model the process of critical reflection. When students provide evidence of their ways of understanding, through either written reflective tasks or verbal structured feedback about their learning, this represents, from the perspective of critical reflection theories, a valid and valuable source of knowledge, and has implications for how students' reflections are used and acted upon within the curriculum. Students are encouraged to move fluidly and iteratively between theory and practice knowledge, and are exposed to the tangible outcomes of critical reflection where the knowledge gained and communicated, through their critical reflections on learning, is used to inform curriculum development.

Figure 1.2 illustrates how the underpinning theories of reflexivity, postmodernism and critical theory facilitate students to engage in critical reflection tasks. The knowledge arising from students' reflective activity informs the curriculum, including the setting

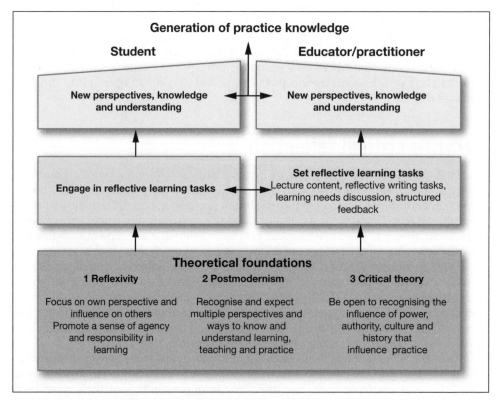

Figure 1.2 Theoretical foundations informing practice knowledge

and refinement of reflective tasks, and the bi-directional arrows between students and educators reflect that both parties benefit from participating in set reflective tasks.

Using the iterative model of critical reflection as a comparison, studies that analyse the content of students' reflections on the basis of the themes raised or the level of reflection demonstrated, might be missing a vital point of critical reflection. Being critically reflective about knowledge and experience means valuing a range of perspectives and being prepared to act on such knowledge to change teaching or learning practices. For example, Chur-Hansen (2008) suggests that one of the most valuable teaching and learning outcomes from ongoing examination of students' portfolio writing was the ability of the educator to better understand how and why student learning difficulties arise, as they arise. If students' interpretations and understanding are actively and visibly incorporated into the process of curriculum development, students are provided with a practical example of the value of being critical in what they offer because of the inherent value that their contributions are given.

Opportunities for this exchange of knowledge and interpretation occur during individual educator–student feedback sessions where educators should take seriously information that students provide and incorporate it, as far as practically possible, in guiding the next learning opportunity (see Fig 1.2). Themes that emerge from students' reflective writing should be used as both a source of knowledge to inform other students who may experience similar learning events, and to inform curriculum content and pedagogy.

We argue that critical reflection tasks are not an end in themselves but, by understanding the theoretical platform upon which they are based, incorporating critical reflection into the curriculum provides a means for educators to iteratively move between the theories of knowledge about learning that students provide, and their task of designing educational opportunities that respond to and nurture student learning. Taking perspectives and interpretations seriously is a key step when critically analysing experiences. This is no less important when educators set critical reflection tasks for students.

Implementing iterative critical reflection: vertical integration in a four-year physiotherapy course

In this section, we provide an overview of how the theories of critical reflection and the associated tasks are introduced in a four-year undergraduate physiotherapy program at Monash University in Australia. There are two key tenets of the iterative model of critical reflection that have been incorporated into this program. The first is the importance of exposing students to underpinning theory in critical reflection. We argue that students need access to concepts and language in order to achieve the objectives of the reflective tasks set for them. The second is that in the early stages of clinical practice, students are encouraged and provided with the skills to move out of 'pure description' into critical analysis and the use of theories to generate strategies for improved learning and practice.

Critical reflection theories and tasks: vertical integration in an undergraduate physiotherapy curriculum

In the first two years of the undergraduate program, the critical reflection curriculum was designed to encourage students to reflect on their own knowledge, and to recognise and distinguish between their personal frames of reference and the new knowledge and ideas introduced in lectures, case-based discussion groups and practical classes. Supporting lectures focused on reflexivity as an underlying theory of critical reflection. The first critical reflection assignment required students to identify learning incidents from practical classes, personal lectures or case-based learning groups, and to reflect on the influence of different domains of knowledge including propositional, professional craft knowledge and their own personal knowledge (Higgs & Titchen 2000). The associated guidelines for this written assignment were to provide:

1 A very brief description of what occurred; that is, a learning experience(s) or session(s) that you particularly remember.
2 An analysis of the event:
   - how it influenced your understanding of professionalism
   - the influence of different domains of knowledge
   - a description of personal feelings and responses
   - an explanation of what sense was made of the personal feelings and responses, and of the personal 'lessons learnt'
   - a statement of how the 'lessons learnt' will influence future actions, professional development and continued learning.

Students were advised that there was no correct answer, and that both positive and negative aspects of the feelings and responses would be acknowledged. Other writing and interactive tasks that incorporated critical reflection in the first two years included self and peer evaluation of their practical skills via a structured skills mastery session, and case-based learning discussion that emphasised giving and receiving feedback as a form of (peer-based) critical reflection.

In the second two years, when students spent more time in clinical placements, the focus shifted from facilitating skills of self-awareness to providing students with theories and tasks that enabled them to recognise and understand multiple perspectives in the less structured and more complex clinical setting. The two supporting critical reflection lectures provided underlying theories about critical theory, postmodernism and qualitative research methodologies. The first lecture introduced critical theory as an approach to analysing students' personal learning styles, and an analysis of how individual perspectives and methods of learning may be affected by the student–supervisor relationship, the hierarchical structure of hospital settings, and the perspectives of other healthcare colleagues. The second lecture outlined theories of postmodermism and linked the ideas of multiple perspectives to ways of understanding patients' histories, experiences, personal perspectives and interests within the context of clinical interviews.

The associated critical reflection task was in the form of an essay about a critical incident or a series of events that students encountered in their clinical placements. Students were given explicit instructions about 'critical' thinking and writing in the form of marking criteria (Table 1.1). These criteria guided the students to move iteratively between theories that could explain their critical incident, and their personal reactions and interpretations of the learning experience or clinical experiences.

Other writing tasks included interviewing, recording, transcribing and analysing a single interview with a patient (with university research ethics approval). The aim of the interview and subsequent analysis was to explore the beliefs, perspectives and experiences of health and wellbeing for a person. To guide their analysis and writing, students attended lectures on qualitative analysis of written transcripts; theories of postmodernism and critical theory; and methods of critical analysis and writing.

In the fourth year of the program, students' critical reflection tasks were integrated closely with their clinical skill acquisition. Interactions with clinical supervisors were used to facilitate students' critical thinking and expression. For example, at the beginning

GRADE	HOW DOES THE WRITING DEMONSTRATE LINKING OF THEORY TO PRACTICE APPROPRIATE TO THE STUDENTS' AREA OF LEARNING?	HOW DOES THE WRITING DEMONSTRATE THE USE OF RESOURCES AND THEIR APPLICATION?	WHAT LEVEL OF CRITICAL REFLECTION, USING ANALYSIS, SYNTHESIS AND EVALUATION DOES THE WRITING DEMONSTRATE?
80–100%	1 Challenges personal assumptions through structured reflection on own and others' practice 2 Critically discusses relevant cultural, ethical and professional issues 3 Analyses potential for discrimination within the situation	1 Locates and accesses an extensive range of relevant sources of information	1 Critically analyses experiences and practices 2 Demonstrates breadth in their reflective writing, including the development of both sensible and insightful ways to think about their learning experiences 3 Explores new approaches based on reflection of personal experiences and other sources of knowledge 4 Articulates clear and relevant arguments and discussions about their experiences 5 Demonstrates independent, insightful and logical conclusions
70–80%	1 Challenges personal assumptions through reflection on own and others' practice 2 Explores relevant cultural, ethical and professional issues 3 Recognises potential for discrimination within the situation	1 Locates and accesses a range of relevant sources of information 2 Evaluates validity of information	1 Begins to develop views, ideas and approaches that may help to offer new knowledge 2 Demonstrates the development of both sensible and insightful ways to think about their learning experiences 3 Highlights new approaches based on reflection of personal experiences and other sources of knowledge 4 Articulates arguments and discussions about their experiences 5 Demonstrates some independent, insightful and logical conclusions
60–70%	1 Describes and reflects on own practice 2 Considers cultural, ethical and professional issues	1 Locates and accesses an adequate range of relevant information	1 Begins to demonstrate critical thinking and analysis of practice and literature in a straightforward manner 2 Demonstrates a limited range of problem identification and problem solving ability 3 Develops some arguments, using appropriate sources, and draws simplistic conclusions
50–60%	1 Limited reflection on practice 2 Limited consideration of relevant cultural, ethical or professional issues	1 Locates and accesses a limited range of relevant information	1 Demonstrates limited critical thinking 2 Describes relevant arguments without evaluation 3 Assembles and links ideas from a limited range of sources 4 Draws some relevant conclusions
Below 50	1 Demonstrates insufficient reflection on practice 2 Insufficient consideration of relevant cultural ethical or professional issues	1 Locates and accesses irrelevant or insufficient information	1 Provides a purely descriptive account throughout 2 Lacks evidence of ability for critical thinking 3 Presents random points and weak arguments 4 Presents inadequate conclusions

Table 1.1 Criteria for marking critical reflection essay (adapted from Shutz et al 2004, p 63)

of each placement students were required to meet with their clinical educator to discuss their learning needs for the particular clinical placement. To facilitate students' critical analysis of their learning needs, they were required to complete a 'learning needs' form (Fig 1.3). Successful completion of this form required a high level of collaboration and critical analysis of strengths and weaknesses in both learning and teaching skills.

In the final section of this chapter, we provide an extended excerpt from one student's third year critical reflection essay. In order to evaluate both the content and level of critical analysis, we obtained ethics approval and the consent of the students to de-identify their essays, and to analyse them for themes raised about clinical placement experiences and their level of critical analysis. Themes to emerge from analysis of the reflective essay content are listed in Table 1.2.

Dealing with death and dying was the most prevalent theme raised by students. The second most frequent topic was negotiating professional relationships with patients, clinical educators or other healthcare professionals. This theme is prominent in the excerpt below from the student we have called Sally. Sally's writing style and content is representative of the 53 students (82% of the total year level) who provided their informed consent to de-identify and make a copy of their essays. The essay excerpt provides an in-depth example of the process of critical reflection and, in particular, how the student identifies theoretical perspectives to guide new knowledge and increase her understanding of the learning incident.

Sally's critical reflection essay excerpt

EVENT: DESCRIPTION—WHAT HAPPENED

In the 13th week of my placement, I was introduced to a new patient (a 52-year-old female) for whom I was to complete a subjective and objective assessment. I learnt the patient had recently undergone a right total hip replacement. The patient explained that she suffered from anxiety and was grieving the loss of her husband who had lost his battle with mesothelioma earlier in the year.

When I asked the patient about falls history, she revealed that her late husband had been physical in the years before he was sick and occasionally pushed her around, one time pushing her to the ground where she sustained a hair line fracture to her right wrist and some broken ribs. I immediately asked the patient if she had spoken to anyone about her grief and past experiences, and she explained she had been seeing a grief counsellor and she was aware she had access to the clinical psychologist from the hospital should she require his expertise.

Throughout the physical examination, the patient required constant reassurance that everything was as it should be with her hip. She was extremely anxious and concerned about doing something that could damage her hip, and really nervous about coping at home on her own. She explained that earlier this morning she felt she sat down too quickly in the chair in her room and was worried she may have dislocated her hip. The patient asked me to check numerous times that her legs were the same length, both today and the other 15 days of her stay.

REACTION

I experienced overwhelming feelings of sympathy for this patient and all she had been through, which is why I had such a hard time understanding that after the first few days of treating her, I really began to dread seeing her. I felt drained, and began resenting her constant need for reassurance. This made me feel so terrible because I didn't want to be uncaring and I had never experienced these feelings with a patient before. I was never rude or short with the patient, but there were times when I just felt like screaming, 'You are fine. Stop asking me the same things about your recovery. You are

Clinical placement
Learning needs form

This form should be completed at the beginning of each of your clinical placements or whenever you change supervisors. Completing this form and discussing it with your clinical educator helps to facilitate effective learning and effective learning relationships.

1   What are you expecting to learn in this clinic?

2   Identify strengths and weaknesses in each of the following areas of learning:
   - Theoretical knowledge
   - Skills-communication/assessment/treatment
   - Attitudes/motivation/interest

3   Learning style
   - Identify your dominant or preferred learning style

4   Feedback
   - What are your views about receiving feedback?
   - What steps can you and your clinical educator(s) take to make feedback helpful for your learning?

5   English fluency
   - Do you translate questions in English to another language?
   - Do you have any concerns about English fluency on this clinic?

6   What are your learning goals and how can these goals be best facilitated in this clinic?

Learning goal	Student actions or learning strategies	Educator actions or teaching strategies

Figure 1.3 Learning needs form

THEMES RAISED IN STUDENTS' CRITICAL INCIDENTS	STUDENTS WHO FOCUSED ON THEME
Death and dying	28%
Professional relationships	23%
Receiving feedback	9%
Clinical reasoning	8%
Ethics	8%
Patient-centred care	6%
Assessing and treating patients with neurological conditions	6%
Student anxiety about their beginner practitioner status	5%
Other	7%

Table 1.2 Themes raised by students in their critical reflections on clinical education (*n* = 53)

much better off than most of the people in here and you'll manage perfectly well when you go home.'

After these thoughts I'd feel an enormous amount of guilt knowing what she had been through in the past couple of years and knowing she was aware of her anxieties, which often resulted in her apologising to me for her constant need for reassurance. I also felt angry at myself for feeling this way especially as I was surrounded by healthcare professionals that had been treating patients for so many years, and here was me after 13 weeks, thinking it was all too much. I did begin to wonder if I was just tired and stressed from the whole clinical experience, and began questioning my abilities to cope when I was confronted with patients and situations I found difficult in the 'clinical world'.

The bad thing about the experience was feeling like I was an unkind person for experiencing feelings of frustration with this patient. It was good however for me to learn that I was not alone in having these kinds of reactions towards a patient, and that it is important to debrief to someone about these feelings before they manifest into something serious like compassion fatigue.

ANALYSIS: MAKING SENSE OF THE EXPERIENCE

On Tuesday, one week after meeting this patient, I attended a tutorial run by the physiotherapy department especially designed for student de-briefing and reflection. The topic of the tutorial was compassion fatigue, a topic I could really relate to at this time of my placement.

Compassion fatigue (CF) is a phenomenon often experienced by healthcare professions that deal with patients who have undergone physical and emotional trauma. It occurs when a caregiver becomes overwhelmed with repeat empathetic contact with a patient. It can present with both psychological and physiological symptoms, such as withdrawal, task avoidance, anger, frustration, sadness, irritability and sleep disturbance (Figley 2002). Some of the reasons CF is prevalent among healthcare workers include employment in settings with a number of patients that have experienced trauma, bi-demand work environment due to decreased resources often resulting in multi-tasking and the difficulty separating empathy and objectivity with patients (Kraus 2006).

Compassion fatigue is not only detrimental to the psychological and physiological state of the healthcare provider but can also lead to a poor quality of healthcare received by the patient (Worley 2005). Carers suffering from CF often detach themselves from their patients rather than engaging with them, and Huggard (2003) describes reasons for this detachment may include preventing themselves from 'burning out' or becoming physically and mentally exhausted, to help improve their concentration and to help improve their own time management.

As well as the impact CF has on the individual, White (2006) outlines the impact CF can have on the workplace. Employees who may be experiencing CF symptoms may exhibit decreased productivity with increased time off, difficulties managing their role in the workplace and reduced morale. This in turn leads to increased workloads for other employees and reduced quality of care for patients.

It is important to note, while there is a lot of literature available on the phenomenon of CF, there was no literature that specifically discussed CF among physiotherapists or physiotherapy students.

ACTION: IF IT AROSE AGAIN, WHAT I WOULD DO DIFFERENTLY

Having reflected on the thoughts and feelings I experienced when treating this patient, and the content of the tutorial which enlightened me with an understanding of CF, I know if I was in a similar situation again, I would definitely find someone to talk to about the way I was feeling.

Thankfully I was in a situation where my patient's quality of care and my own wellbeing were not compromised, but having been introduced to the concept of CF has just made me aware that it is something that can happen to physiotherapists in the nature of the work we do.

Some self-management suggestions for people affected by CF were outlined in an article by Pfifferling and Gilley (2000), and I have included them as possible plans of action. Find someone to talk to, understand the thoughts and feelings you have are normal, start exercising and eating properly, get enough sleep, take some time off, develop interests outside your line of work and identify what's important to you.

I have developed a firm respect for the importance of critical reflection. Writing my thoughts and feelings down for each week was a very therapeutic task for me and really helped me contemplate my worries and concerns. It outlined what was important to me in relation to my interactions with patients and interactions with my supervisor and the multi-disciplinary team.

Sally's writing illustrates a number of the features of the iterative critical reflection model. The strongest feature of her writing is the way she incorporated the idea of reflexivity. Sally acknowledges and appreciates the influence of herself (her relative lack of experience, her behavioural and emotional reactions) and importantly, her sense of self or agency in having a role in influencing another person. Through the process of reflexively locating herself in this experience, Sally's analysis leads her to identify new knowledge and ways of coping with her reactions of guilt and frustration. Sally's reflexively also leads her to a new sense and understanding of the broader responsibilities associated with health practice. Notions of patient dependency, providing non-clinical advice, and recognising limitations are all themes raised by Sally's reflection and, importantly, are integrated into writing about future action.

Sally also refers explicitly to theories of knowledge about 'compassion fatigue' in healthcare work as a way to account for her own reactions, and she moves from that theory back to her own experience to suggest ways she might act in the future, including making a list of tips for practice for future students. Using the more formalised theory and explanations of CF, she is able to theorise her experience and, in so doing, builds for herself a broader and more generalised theory about how to manage this type of clinical experience in the future.

Although Sally does not name specific critical theories, her tips for future students illustrate an implicit understanding of the influence of power differences between clinical educators and students, and she urges future students to 'be strong about asking for feedback' and seeking support (see Table 1.3).

Don't expect as a student, a grade one or even a senior clinician that you are going to know everything. Physiotherapy is a career of life-long learning. Embrace what you don't know, don't look at it as a negative thing.
Be strong about asking for feedback. If you don't feel you are receiving the feedback you need, let your supervisor know. If this doesn't change, then speak to someone (perhaps head of the department or university). You have the right to receive adequate feedback about your performance.
Prepare yourself each day. Before going to bed, write a list of what you plan to do for the next day. I felt this helped me sleep and stopped me worrying I was not organised.
Try to enjoy yourself. We are privileged to have such an intense clinical experience as physiotherapy students, and placements gives us the opportunity to determine what areas of physio we are really interested in and to practise the skills we have been working so hard to learn.

Table 1.3 Tips and strategies arising from a critical reflection essay

Sally's writing provides an example of how critical reflection that moves iteratively between theories explaining learning events can be transformatory in nature, and inculcate a culture of searching for solutions and new understanding as a feature of healthcare practice. Finally, her writing illustrates important features of the method of the critical reflection process, previously identified by Pease and Fook (1999, p 200):

1 An ability to recognise and appreciate the influences of behavioural and emotional reactions, background and experience.
2 An ability to identify personally held assumptions and to acknowledge how these assumptions influence reactions and understanding of experience.
3 A sense of responsibility or agency about one's ability to influence experience or change an outcome.
4 A capacity to accept uncertainty as part of learning and health practice, and to use uncertainty as a catalyst to seek and develop new knowledge and understanding.

Modelling iterative critical reflection

In addition to vertically integrating theories and tasks of critical reflection into the undergraduate curricula for students, we also advocate the importance of modelling 'transformative' reflective practice, where insights from students, academics and clinical staff are translated into pragmatic curricula or institutional changes. This form of modelling where learners can see the links between inquiry, critical thinking and change, is essential in helping shape students' construction of reflection as part of practice, rather than a metacognitive add-on to their learning in clinical practice. Modelling of reflective practice can be expressed through the transparent modification of the academic curriculum arising from student and educator feedback. It can also be modelled via individual university-based and clinical educators demonstrating skills in reflective thinking.

For example, in their reflective essay task in third year, the theme of death and dying was raised by many students. This topic was subsequently introduced into the curriculum in the final undergraduate year through the introduction of a lecture and a case-based learning scenario centred on palliative care. The theme of negotiating relationships was addressed through the inclusion of a 'non-technical skills' session in the pre-clinical transition week. This involved students being given opportunities to practise skills of negotiation with simulated or standardised patients. Example scenarios included presenting at a multi-disciplinary team meeting, breaking bad news, and engaging in one-to-one feedback with the clinical educator. Finally, the tips for future practice written by each student as a component of their essay were collated and used directly to inform the development of the curriculum for the next student cohort.

Acting on themes and tips presented in student essays is more than collecting feedback about student learning. We believe that transparently using student reflection is a form of iterative reflection about educational practice. Moving between student insight, knowledge and evaluation, and development of educational content and teaching methods reflects our underpinning theoretical stance on reflective practice. That is, that reflective practice is not just about 'contemplation and analysis' but also about transformative change. The model of reflection advocated in this chapter moves beyond 'the swampy lowlands' of reflection-on and in-practice as advocated by Schön (1987) in his account of reflection in professional practice. Rather, we emphasise the importance of using the theoretical underpinnings of critical reflection to inform critical reflection activities. The important underlying assumption in this approach is that valuing and explaining a philosophical frame of reference is key when learning requires an ability to adapt to new, and potentially ambiguous, situations (Brawer 2006, Higgs et al 2004).

Although we have relied on the evaluation of the quality of students' written reflection essays as a surrogate indicator of the effectiveness of our program, the actual translation and effect in clinical practice of learning these reflective skills through writing and feedback tasks is unknown. Ongoing research is required to assess whether the iterative model of critical reflection introduced in the academic program translates to skills in clinical practice.

Conclusion

In this chapter we have presented a model of iterative critical reflection, characterised by moving between description and analysis of healthcare practice and underpinning explanatory theories of critical reflection. We argue that for students to develop habits of critical reflection in their professional practice, they must be exposed to explicit teaching of reflective practice principles and theories, along with modelling of critical reflection by university and clinically based educators.

We suggest that by making transparent to students the transformative nature of reflective practice, through listening to students' recommendations and acting on these recommendations, that reflection is conceptualised as a key *part of practice* rather than positioned as a retrospective metacognitive activity. In presenting our iterative model of critical reflection, we hope to promote a deeper understanding of how skills in critical reflection might be meaningfully incorporated into health professional education.

References

Baird M, Winter J 2005 Reflection, practice and clinical education. In: Rose M, Best D (eds) Best transforming practice through clinical education, professional supervision and mentoring. Elsevier, Edinburgh

Barry C, Britten N, Barber N et al 1999 Using reflexivity to optimise teamwork in qualitative research. Qualitative Health Research 9(1):26–44

Bleakley A 2006 Broadening conceptions of learning in medical education: the message from team working. Medical Education 40:150–157

Boenink A, Oderwald A, De Jonge P, Van Tilberg W, Smal J 2004 Assessing student reflection in medical practice. The development of an observer-rated instrument: reliability, validity and initial experiences. Medical Education 38:368–377

Boud D 1993 Experience as the base for learning. Higher education research and development 12(1):33–44

Boud D, Keogh R, Walker D 1985 Reflection: Turning experience into learning. Kogan Page, London

Brawer JR 2006 The value of a philosophical perspective in teaching the basic medical sciences. Medical Teacher 28(5):472–474

Brookfield S 1995 Becoming a critically reflective teacher. Jossey-Bass, San Francisco

Chirema K 2007 The use of reflective journals in the promotion of reflection and learning in post-registration nursing students. Nurse Education Today 27:192–202

Chur-Hansen A 2008 Keeping a journal of reflections on learning. In: Facione N, Facione P Critical thinking and clinical reasoning in the health sciences: An international multidisciplinary teaching anthology. California Academic Press, Millbrae, California

Clouder L 2000 Reflective practice: realising its potential. Physiotherapy 86(10):517–522

Cole K, Barker R, Kolodner K et al 2004 Faculty development in teaching skills: An intensive longitudinal model. Academic Medicine: 5(May): 469–480

Cross V 1993 Introducing physiotherapy students to the idea of 'reflective practice'. Medical Teacher 15(4):293–307

Cross V 1997 The Professional Development Diary: a case study of one cohort of physiotherapy students. Physiotherapy Research Report 83(7):375–383

Delany C, Watkin D 2008 A study of critical reflection in health professional education: 'Learning where others are coming from'. Advances in Health Sciences Education. Online. Available: www.springerlink.com/content/v05423601p317432/ Accessed 8 Jan 2008

Dewey J 1933 How we think: a restatement of the relation of reflective thinking to the educative process. DC Heath, Massachusetts

Dornan T, Boshuizen H, King N et al 2007 Experience-based learning: a model linking processes and outcomes of medical students' workplace learning. Medical Education 41:84–91

Driessen EW et al 2005 Conditions for successful reflective use of portfolios in undergraduate medical education. Medical Education 39:1230–1235

Driscoll J 2000 Practising clinical supervision: a reflective approach. Bailliere Tindall, Edinburgh

Dye D 2005 Enhancing critical reflection of students during a clinical internship using the SOAP note. The internet Journal of Allied Health Sciences and Practice 3(4)

Edwards I, Jones M, Carr J et al 2004 Clinical reasoning strategies in physical therapy. Physical Therapy 84(4):312–330

Ende J, Pomerantz A, Erickson F 1995 Preceptors' strategies for correcting residents in an ambulatory care medicine setting: A qualitative analysis. Academic Medicine 70:224–229

Eraut M 1994 Developing professional knowledge and competence. Falmer, London

Figley C 2002 Compassion fatigue: psychotherapists' chronic lack of self-care. Psychotherapy in Practice 58(11):1433–1441

Fook J 2002 Theorising from practice: Towards an inclusive approach for social work. Qualitative Social Work 1(1):79–95

Fook J 2004 Critical reflection and transformative possibilities. In: Davies L, Leonard P (eds) Social work in a corporate era: practices of power and resistance. Ashgate, Aldershot, UK

Francis D 1995 The reflective journal: a window to pre-service teachers' practical knowledge. Teaching & teacher education 11:229–241

Frye A, Hollingsworth M, Wymer A, Hinds A 1997 A qualitative study of faculty techniques for giving feedback to interns following an observed standardised patient encounter. In: Scherpbier A, van der Vleuten C, Rethans J, van der Steeg A (eds) Advances in medical education. Kluwer Academic, Dordrecht, 216–219

Gardner F 2003 Critical reflection in community-based evaluation. Qualitative Social Work 2(2):197–212

Gibbs G 1988 Learning by doing: a guide to teaching and learning methods. Oxford Brookes University, Oxford

Guillemin M, Gillam L 2004 Ethics, reflexivity and 'ethically important moments' in research. Qualitative Enquiry 10(2):261–280

Hansen E 2006 Successful qualitative health research. Allen & Unwin, Sydney

Hatton N, Smith D 1995 Reflection in teacher education: Towards definition and implementation. Teaching and Teacher Education 11(1):33–49

Henderson P, Ferguson-Smith A, Johnson M 2005 Developing essential professional skills: a framework for teaching and learning about feedback. Biomed Central Medical Education 5

Henderson P, Johnson M 2002 An innovative approach to developing the reflective skills of medical students. Biomed Central Medical Education 2:4

Herbert R, Jamtvedt G, Mead J et al 2005 Practical evidence-based physiotherapy. Elsevier, Edinburgh

Higgs J, Andresen L, Fish D 2004 Practice knowledge: Its nature, sources and contexts. In: Higgs J, Richardson B, Dahlgren M (eds) Developing practice knowledge. Butterworth-Heinemann, Edinburgh

Higgs J, Titchen A 2000 Knowledge and reasoning. In: Higgs J, Jones M (eds) Clinical reasoning in the health professions, 2nd edn. Butterworth-Heinemann, New York

Higgs J, Titchen A 2001 Rethinking the practice–knowledge interface in an uncertain world: A model for practice development. British Journal of Occupational Therapy 64(11):526–533

Howell J 1989 The reflective practitioner in nursing. Journal of Advanced Nursing 14:824–832

Huggard P 2003 Compassion fatigue: how much can I give? Medical Education 37:163–164

Iedema R, Degeling P, Braithwaite J et al 2004 Medical education and curriculum reform: putting reform proposals in context. Medical Education Online 9(17) Available: www.med-ed-online.org/f0000091.htm Accessed 9 Jan 2009

Jensen G 2005 Mindfulness: Applications for teaching and learning in ethics education. In: Purtilo R, Jensen G, Brasic Royeen C (eds) Educating for moral action, FA Davis, Philadelphia

Jensen GM, Gwyer J, Shepard KF et al 2000 Expert practice in physical therapy. Physical Therapy 80:28–43

Jensen G, Shepard K, Hack L 1990 The novice versus the experienced clinician: insights into the work of the physical therapist. Physical Therapy 70(5):314–323

Johns C 1995 Framing learning through reflection within Carper's fundamental ways of knowing in nursing. Journal of Advanced Nursing 22:226–234

Kember D 2001 Reflective Teaching and learning in the health professions. Blackwell Science, Oxford

Kneebone R 2002 Total internal reflection: an essay on paradigms. Medical Education 36:514–518

Kraus C 2006 Compassion fatigue: what is it, and how can you avoid it? Alabama Nurse 32(4):18

Larin H, Wessel J, Al-Shamlan A 2005 Reflections of physiotherapy students in the United Arab Emirates during their clinical placements: A qualitative study. Biomed Central Medical Education 5(3)

McLeod S, Romanini J, Cohn E et al 1997 Models and roles in clinical education. In: McAllister L, Lincoln M, Mcleod S, Maloney D (eds) Facilitating learning in clinical settings. Stanley Thornes, Cheltenham, UK

Maudsley G, Strivens J 2000 Promoting professional knowledge, experiential learning and critical thinking for medical students. Medical Education 34:535–544

Mezirow J 1991 Transformative dimensions of adult learning. Jossey Bass, San Francisco

Molloy E, Clarke D 2005 The positioning of physiotherapy students and clinical supervisors in feedback sessions. Focus on health professional education: a multi-disciplinary journal 7:79–90

Patton M 2002 Qualitative research and evaluation methods, 3rd edn. Sage, California

Pease R, Fook J 1999 Postmodern critical theory and emancipatory social work practice. In: Pease R, Fook J (eds) Transforming social work practice. Routledge, London, 1–22

Pee B, Wodman T, Fry H et al 2002 Appraising and assessing reflection in students' writing on a structured worksheet. Medical Education 36:575–585

Pfifferling J, Gilley K 2000 Overcoming compassion fatigue. Family Practice Management 7(4):39–44

Rees C 2004 The problem with outcomes-based curricula in medical education: insights from educational theory. Medical Education 38:593–598

Rice P, Ezzy D 1999 Qualitative research methods: A health focus. Oxford University Press, Oxford

Richardson G, Maltby H 1995 Reflection-on-practice: enhancing student learning. Journal of Advanced Nursing 22:235–242

Rose M, Best D (eds) 2005 Transforming practice through clinical education, professional supervision and mentoring. Elsevier, Edinburgh

Routledge J, Willson M, McArthur M et al 1997 Reflection on the development of a reflective assessment. Medical Teacher 19(2):122–128

Ryan S, Esdaile S, Brown G 2003 Appreciating the big picture: you are part of it! In: Brown G, Esdaile S, Ryan S (eds) Becoming an advanced healthcare practitioner. Butterworth Heinemann, Edinburgh, 1–29

Schön D 1983 The reflective practitioner: how professionals think in action. Basic Books, New York

Schön D 1987 Educating the beginning practitioner. Jossey-Bass, San Francisco

Schutz S, Angove C, Sharp P 2004 Assessing and evaluating reflection. In: Bulman C, Shutz S (eds) Reflective practice in nursing. Blackwell, Oxford

Shepard K, Hack L, Gwyer J, Jensen G 1999 Describing expert practice in physical therapy. Qualitative Health Research 9(6):746–758

Snadden D, Thomas M 1998 The use of portfolio learning in medical education. Medical Teacher 20:192–199

Talbot M 2004 Monkey see, monkey do: a critique of the competency model in graduate medical education. Medical Education 38:587–592

Taylor C, White S 2000 Practicing reflexivity in health and welfare. Buckingham, Philadelphia

Trede F, Higgs J, Jones M et al 2003 Emancipatory practice: a model for physiotherapy practice. Focus on health professional education: A multidisciplinary journal 5(2):1–13

Wessel J, Larin H 2006 Change in reflections of physiotherapy students over time in clinical placements. Learning in Health & Social Care 5(3):119–132

White D 2006 The hidden costs of caring: what managers need to know. The Health Care Manager 25(4):341–347

Worley C 2005 The art of caring: compassion fatigue. Dermatology Nursing 17:6

CHAPTER 2

Ways of knowing for clinical practice

Joy Higgs

THEORIES

Sociocultural and historical constructions of knowledge provide the key theoretical perspectives underpinning this chapter. They are used to enhance increased understanding of past and future directions in education practice.

USING THEORIES TO INFORM CURRICULUM DESIGN AND RESEARCH

When reviewing and designing clinical education curricula, it is important to provide opportunities for students to consider how their practice and professional knowledge is historically derived and how it intersects with aspects of the sociocultural environment in which they will practise. A key underlying premise of clinical education curricula is the understanding of knowledge; its construction, context and use in practice.

USING THEORIES TO DRIVE EDUCATION METHODS

Example: Practical ways to incorporate sociocultural theories of knowledge construction include ensuring that students are prompted to consider what constitutes their practice knowledge; how their professional knowledge is created and developed; and how practitioners, researchers and educators contribute to ways of knowing and practicing as a health professional. For example, in practical–clinical skills sessions students could be asked to consider the justification for applying a particular treatment method, and they should be expected to have a broad and inclusive understanding of the evidence to support clinical practice. Focusing on the historical development and sociocultural influences on professional ways of practicing provides a means of enhancing and broadening students' understanding of their own learning experiences.

Introduction

A key goal of clinical education is to foster the development of the learner's knowledge base. The first task in pursuing this goal is to understand the nature of knowledge. In this chapter knowledge is presented as a sociocultural, historical construction embedded in the language, discourse and practice of the setting and time in which it is used. This is illustrated by several examples of how knowledge has been influenced, along with practice, by changes in political, social, educational and cultural circumstances in different eras. It is argued that a deeper understanding of the way knowledge is constructed and used in practice is essential for good practice and for sound clinical education. The importance of making explicit our practice epistemology (i.e. the knowledge and ways of knowing underpinning practice) in practice and education is a key argument presented in this chapter and in previous work (Higgs et al 2008c, Richardson et al 2004). See also Chapter 1 of this book where knowing and learning in social frameworks is discussed.

History, practice, education and knowledge

History provides us with an understanding of the way current practice and knowledge has emerged and the factors influencing this development. Education of health professionals has both responded and contributed to this evolution. In particular, clinical education has played an important part in the shaping of practice knowledge and knowledge of what it means to be a health professional. In considering the origins and evolving influences on the nature of professional practice and education in the health sciences Higgs and Hunt (1999) identified the following stages in this evolution.

a   The apprentice

Traditional healthcare workers operated and learned in an apprenticeship model. They learned in the workplace setting, studied the master's art, progressed through simple, highly supervised tasks to more complex and independent tasks, became independent practitioners and, potentially, masters themselves. The apprenticeship system focused on the practice knowledge, craft and art, and the practical role of the healthcare worker. The quality of this system ranged from poor, with unquestioned or required adoption of ill-founded practices and knowledge reflected by poor role models, to excellent, where the apprentice learned from expert role models who offered individual, knowledgeable tuition, direct demonstration and quality supervision. Such education persisted for many years in hospital-based programs (Twomey 1980) and early tertiary education programs, where knowledge of experienced practitioner educators was passed on, rather uncritically, to the next generation. The main concern with this approach is the limitation of the novice's development to the mentor's level of expertise.

b   The health professional

Traditionally, established professions such as medicine have owned a body of knowledge, operated in a service mode under a code of professional conduct, and sought to establish the quality of performance through self-regulation. The professionalisation of other health disciplines in the first half of the twentieth century involved the desire to attain professional status and credibility, the pursuit of professional attributes and (commonly) the adoption of the medical model along with justification of the discipline's professional knowledge and skills through (medical) scientific research and priorities. The model of practice adopted was one of professional activity comprising instrumental problem solving, made rigorous by the use of scientific theory and technique. Educational programs of this era emphasised socialisation into the professional role and the acquisition of the knowledge, skills and attitudes needed to enter the profession as capable beginning practitioners.

c   The clinical problem solver

Learning to cope with the knowledge and technology explosions and the threat of rapid knowledge obsolescence in the second half of the twentieth century saw an increased emphasis on the skills of problem solving, with a diminishing emphasis on knowledge acquisition. For some, this cognitive skill orientation was over-emphasised and the reliance on problem-solving skills in the absence of a sound knowledge base was criticised. Research in the area of clinical reasoning and problem solving (Norman 1988), for instance, supported the essential link between knowledge and reasoning, while Boshuizen and Schmidt (1992, 1995) identified the importance of concurrent development of domain-specific knowledge and cognitive skills to use this knowledge as part of the process of developing clinical reasoning expertise. (See Chapter 4.)

d   The competent clinician

In the 1970s and 1980s much interest was generated in competencies (principally technical skills, but later also cognitive and interpersonal skills and the capacity to learn, conduct research and self-evaluate). In many cases, competency-based education led to an atomistic approach to education and practice rather than a holistic approach of caring for the whole person. As a result of current trends of increased accountability, professional malpractice and government regulation, competencies have become popular again in some arenas. While regulatory influences still emphasise the measurable aspects of competencies, educational advancement has led to the broadening definition of competencies including higher level, generic and person-centred competencies with a greater, but still incomplete, capacity to portray the complex, interactive nature of professional practice.

e   The reflective practitioner

Schön's (1983) model of the reflective practitioner raised concerns about the growing gaps between the practical knowledge and actual competencies required of practitioners in the field and the research-based (propositional) knowledge taught in professional schools. Reflective practice, he argued, was needed to deal with the uncertainty of professional work and workplaces where workers frequently face complex goals and unpredictable ill-defined problems. The reflective practitioner model has attracted both criticism and acclaim. It has certainly provided the impetus for a wider exploration of the nature, importance and scope of reflective practice within client-focused healthcare (e.g. Eraut 1994, Fish & Coles 1998, Fulford et al 1996).

f   The scientist practitioner

The latter part of the twentieth century saw a growing concern with the lack of scientific foundation for aspects of healthcare in both the emerging and the more established health professions. The scientist–practitioner model epitomises a commitment of professional groups to scientific rigour (James 1994) and reflects the escalation of research into the scientific evidence for practice that has characterised recent decades. The global trend of evidence-based practice is encapsulated in Twomey's (1990, p 83) argument that clinicians must be able 'to adequately justify their treatment methods [because] the community demands a high quality of care and a cost-efficient system'.

g   The interactional, person-centred professional

Various models of healthcare and health professional education are emerging in recent decades to counter and broaden the narrow focus in many arenas on the scientific definition of evidence for practice. These models emphasise person-centred care grounded in critical social science principles of emancipatory practice and social responsibility (e.g. Trede & Haynes 2008), and the interactions between health professionals, their partners in healthcare and their environment. Underpinning person-centred healthcare lies a model of practice that supports the emancipation rather than the manipulation of patients. 'Including patients in the decision-making process promises to result in more realistic and appropriate treatments, reduced patient concerns and complaints, and better, sustainable health outcomes, and increased patient and clinician satisfaction' (Trede & Higgs 2003, p 66). A critical approach to thinking and emancipatory knowledge is required for this practice approach. A similar emphasis on people and their relationships is contained in a social ecology model of health practice (and education) introduced by Higgs and Hunt (1999, p 44) which embeds some of the strengths of previous models in the interactivity of social ecology.

> In this model, interactional professionals will be equipped with generic skills (including skills in communication, problem solving, evaluation and investigation, self-directed learning and interpersonal interaction) which will enable them to engage in lifelong learning, research, and professional review and development, as well as in responsible, self-critical autonomous practice of their professional role. They will be capable of interacting effectively with their context in a manner which is transformational, facilitative, interdependent and symbiotic (i.e. both influenced by and influencing that environment). Such individuals will operate within their personal frame of reference and also demonstrate client centredness and credibility in relation to the given situation. They will be competent professionals, interdependent team members, and reflective practitioners capable of substantiation of their actions. Their actions will be those of responsible agents who operate interdependently with people and the environment to address the needs of the situation and to facilitate change for the benefit of their clients and society as a whole.

Table 2.1 summarises these trends and illustrates the powerful interrelationship between knowledge and context.

Knowledge and practice as sociocultural, historical constructions

From the discussion above it is evident that the nature of practice, education and how professional practice knowledge is defined and used are influenced by the sociocultural and historical context of that period of history (see also Larsen et al 2008). Consider, for instance, the following historical influences on practice. In 1986 the World Health Organization's Ottawa Charter (WHO 1986) emphasised the need to develop strategies

CONTEXT	Early traditions of authority and experience	The scientific revolution of the 17th and 18th centuries and the pursuit of professionalisation into the 20th century	20th century knowledge and technology explosions	1970s and 1980s (and recent renewed interest) focus on competencies	1980s, the reflective turn	Late 20th and early 21st century, evidence for practice	Late 20th and early 21st century, quality person-centred care
PRACTICE	Experiential and tradition-led	Medical model dominant in the recognised Western health occupations	Clinical problem solving	Competent practice	Reflective practice	Evidence-based practice	Critical person-centred care
EDUCATION	Apprenticeship	Move to degrees and science-based education of professionals	Problem-based learning	Competency-based education	Educating the reflective practitioner	Teaching scientific evidence for practice	Education for social, service and professional responsibilities
KNOWLEDGE	Experiential and received	Propositional (research and theory driven)	Tools for problem solving	Propositional and technical knowledge	Propositional and non-propositional or experiential knowledge	Propositional knowledge	Propositional and non-propositional or experiential knowledge

Table 2.1 Trends in health professional practice, education and knowledge

'to bring about changes in the physical, social and economic environment in which people live' (Donovan 1995, p 2). One such strategy was to increase the focus on community and environmental health with a greater emphasis on the prevention of disease and the promotion of good health (Higgs et al 1999), as well as the provision of quality acute and chronic healthcare. Lawson et al (1996, p 11) reported a global shift 'away from the cure of individuals presenting for service towards the prevention of illness in populations and the strengthening of the community's capacity to deal with its own health'. In recent years the influence of the communications and information revolution has made an enormous impact on both health practices (e.g. telehealth, and consumer access to self-help information) and the way knowledge is perceived and disseminated. University students, for instance, learn to critically appraise the source and credibility of information widely available on the web.

The context for healthcare in the twenty-first century (Fish & Higgs 2008) encompasses both growing fragmentation and uncertainty, and an unprecedented level of globalisation with increasingly blurred national boundaries, problems of world aid and the complexity of balancing economic demands with decreased public funding resources, all of which have implications for consumers and providers (Higgs et al 1999). Bauman's (2000, 2005) term 'liquid modernity' epitomises the mercurial and unsettled spirit of life in the West in the twenty-first century. Alongside these influences is the 'dot.com mentality' which emphasises short-term abstract fixes rather than long-term relationships with people and, as Sennett (2005) argues, commitment to humane thinking and continuity of care are sidelined. In this age, established knowledge has a short life, and tradition and experience are no longer valued. Fish and Higgs (2008) argue that the 'now', 'same' (cloning) and external scrutiny focus of this age needs to be countered by attention by professionals to being able to present their moral position, to work with 'transparency and integrity, and exercise their clinical thinking and professional judgement in the service of differing individuals, while making wise decisions about the relationship between individuals' privacy and the common good' (p 21). To achieve these outcomes propositional knowledge is inadequate and experiential knowledge (as presented below) is essential, along with changing approaches to what knowledge is and how it is constructed. The rules of the physical sciences knowledge world need to be accompanied by ways of knowing that enable the humanity, nuances and human interests of the social world to be appreciated.

To further illustrate this contextually driven evolution of practice and knowledge consider the example of two professions, physiotherapy and occupational therapy. Pynt et al (2008) discuss the historical antecedents of physiotherapy (such as the use of therapeutic manipulation in ancient Egypt), and the more recent evolution of physiotherapy from the time the occupation gained its identity in Western healthcare to the present time. In their interpretation of the evolution of modern physiotherapy practice, Pynt et al (2008) identify four practice eras.

1 The 'massage era' corresponds to the time frame 1880–1913 and grew out of earlier practice traditions.
2 The 'peripheral neuromusculoskeletal dysfunction era' (1914–1945) was significantly influenced by the poliomyelitis epidemics and World War 1, both of which required the profession to expand its practice and knowledge base to assist in the treatment and management of patients who presented mainly with peripheral neuromusculoskeletal dysfunction.
3 The 'neurological era' occurred during the period 1946 to 1980. Dealing with World War 2 casualties led to the development of rehabilitation practices, the expansion of existing areas of practice such as orthopaedics, and the emergence of new areas,

including plastic surgery and spinal cord injury rehabilitation. The main clinical focus in this era was the management of patients who were affected by dysfunction of the central nervous system (Sahrmann 2002).

4 The 'movement era' (1981–present) reflects the core of contemporary physiotherapy practice, where movement dysfunction is identified as the primary problem addressed by physiotherapy intervention (Sahrmann 2002). The emphasis on movement dysfunction (in the musculoskeletal, neurological, cardiopulmonary and metabolic systems of the human body) is reflected in contemporary definitions of physiotherapy as illustrated by the following extract.

Physical therapy provides services to individuals and populations to develop, maintain and restore maximum movement and functional ability throughout the lifespan. This includes providing services in circumstances where movement and function are threatened by ageing, injury, disease or environmental factors. Functional movement is central to what it means to be healthy. (World Confederation for Physical Therapy 1999, p 1)

Each of these eras saw a progressive and at times dramatic advance in the scientific basis of physiotherapy practice as a consequence of the sociocultural and historical circumstances. The scope of practice expanded and the contributions of the profession to healthcare evolved, along with its knowledge base (Pynt et al 2008).

Occupational therapy is a profession that deals with human occupations. It has undergone a significant evolution in recent decades (Dibden et al 2002). From its early humanistic origins, occupational therapy pursued the legitimation and professionalisation that having a strong association to medicine provided. Recently the profession has reverted to a more community-based orientation compatible with its humanistic origins. This is illustrated in Table 2.2. This journey involved expansion of the profession's knowledge base to include occupational science and practice models and strategies for enhanced consumer involvement in health promotion partnerships.

PERIOD	DEFINITION SUMMARY
Early years	Holistic approach focusing on occupation
1900–60	Medically prescribed treatment using arts and crafts
1960s–70s	Art and science of using activity in health promotion and disability prevention
1970s–90s	Use of purposeful activities to assist individuals attain independence in their daily lives
2000+	Consumer-centred approaches to facilitating meaningful occupation in people's lives

Table 2.2 Evolving patterns in occupational therapy (based on Dibden et al 2002)

In addition to the global changes in practice and knowledge that have occurred across the health professions, and the discipline-specific changes that have characterised the evolution of individual professions as discussed above, knowledge and practice development also occurs at the level of the individual practitioner. Becoming a member of a profession involves professional socialisation including formal and informal education, becoming part of practice communities (including professional groups and workplaces) and individual pursuit of learning and practice development.

Professional socialisation refers to the acculturation process (that occurs through entry education, reflection, professional development and engagement in professional work interactions) by which an individual develops both the expected capabilities of the profession and a sense of professional identity and responsibility. (Higgs et al 2008c, p 59).

Novice practitioners become inducted into communities of professional practice which demand a career-long commitment to meeting the multiple expectations of health professionals set by society, the workplace and the profession in recognition of the privileges of professional status (Higgs et al 2008a). A key expectation relates to the knowledge responsibilities of professionals, including continuing to update one's knowledge and to contribute to the profession's knowledge. This argument is reflected in Cox's (2005) identification of two key features in communities of practice: *situated negotiation of meaning* (which refers to locally and socially constructed knowledge) and *identity being central to learning.* The individual practitioner's knowledge base, the collective knowledge base of a profession and the particular knowledge that defines the practice of both individuals and groups are significant in this learning and identity creation.

Ways of categorising knowledge

A deep interpretation of ways of categorising knowledge is presented by Higgs et al (2008d). This task begins with a recognition that what counts as knowledge is a matter of definition. The definition of knowledge today (Gustavsson 2004) has been significantly influenced by the thinking of Aristotle in the fourth century BC (c.400 BC, 1985 translation) who added to the Platonic concept of *episteme* two further concepts: *techne* and *phronesis.* These three forms of knowledge deal with science, production/creativity and practical wisdom/ethics respectively, and comprise different ways of knowing the physical and human worlds.

A key aspect of categorising knowledge is to recognise how, and in what context, knowledge is generated. A core distinction lies between propositional and non-propositional knowledge. The first includes what Vico (in Berlin 1979) labels deductive (theoretical) knowledge and scientific knowledge (also called empirical knowledge by Carper (1978)). Non-propositional knowledge is also called experiential knowledge (Kolb 1984) and includes Aristotle's *techne* and *phronesis.* Experiential knowledge includes aesthetic, personal and ethical knowing (Carper 1978, Sarter 1988), and professional craft knowledge (gained from professional practice) and personal knowledge (gained from individual and collective life experience) (Higgs & Titchen 1995). (See Table 2.3.)

Practice epistemology

Whether or not practitioners are consciously aware of their practice models and the way they are defining and constructing practice knowledge, they do, in fact, hold views or adopt specific stances or traditions of what counts as legitimate knowledge and what constitutes the domain-specific knowledge of their profession. This is referred to as *practice epistemology.*

Within the biomedical practice framework (or model), for example, with its inherent physical science epistemological stance, knowledge is seen as an objective, predictive, empirical, generalisable, explanatory phenomenon that arises from the use of the natural scientific method and theorisation in a world of external objective reality. In humanistic,

PROPOSITIONAL KNOWLEDGE		NON-PROPOSITIONAL KNOWLEDGE
Research knowledge a The empirico–analytical paradigm produces technical or predictive knowledge where the emphasis is on a cause–effect relationship. b The interpretive paradigm produces practical knowledge that is associated with and embedded in the world of meanings and of human interactions and being. c The critical paradigm produces emancipatory knowledge that deals with how to transform current structures, relationships and conditions which constrain development and reform.	**Theoretical knowledge** Things that are true either by definition or by deduction from propositions or assumptions which are themselves true purely by definition. This knowledge is created through debate and argument.	a Professional craft knowledge can be tacit and is embedded in practice; it comprises general professional knowledge gained from health professionals' practice. b Personal (individual) knowledge includes the collective knowledge held by the community and culture in which the individual lives, and the unique knowledge gained from the individual's life experience.

Table 2.3 Ways of knowing (based on Habermas 1972, Higgs & Titchen 1995)

psychosocial practice models, located in the human and social sciences and the arts, knowledge is seen as being interpretive, theoretical, and constructed in social worlds that recognise and seek to interpret multiple constructed realities. In emancipatory practice models, located in the critical social sciences, knowledge is recognised as being historically and culturally constructed, and historical reality is something that, once understood more deeply, can be changed in order to seek positive changes in practice. (Higgs et al 2008b, p 164)

In 1988 Schön argued that health professionals should proceed beyond the limitations of positivistic views of knowledge, to develop 'an epistemology of practice which places technical problem solving within a broader context of reflective inquiry, shows how reflection-in-action may be rigorous in its own right, and links the art of practice in uncertainty and uniqueness to the scientist's art of research' (Schön 1988, p 60). Eraut, in 1994, contended that higher education institutions should be prepared to extend their roles from 'that of creator and transmitter of generalisable knowledge to that of *enhancing the knowledge creation capacities* of individuals and professional communities' (Eraut 1994, p 57).

In 2004 Higgs et al (p ix) argued:

We are advocating that practice epistemology, or knowing how practice knowledge is created, used and developed (further), should become an explicit dimension of the core, the regularity and the expectation of professional practice. A clear understanding of epistemological beliefs is especially important in the face of the uncertainties inherent in the information revolution and the postmodern world. (This poses four core questions.) … What constitutes practice knowledge? How is this knowledge created and developed? What are the roles of practitioners, researchers and educators, as individuals and members of their communities of practice, in understanding and developing practice knowledge? What are the implications of a practice epistemology model for practice, education and research in the health sciences?

By engaging in a dialogue about these questions with a team of international scholars, practitioners and researchers, these authors reported:

> It is through verbalising their knowledge that practitioners become aware of the strengths and weaknesses of their reasoning and of the claims they make. … Key arguments presented include the importance of reflective practice, the value of peers and practice communities, the need to rethink research and the resulting knowledge for practice, the importance of understanding the nature of practice knowledge, the need to check continually whether professional knowledge is adequate for practice and community needs, the need to recognise the reciprocity between growth and change in practice and knowledge, and the importance of keeping in tune with the information technology revolution (as a tool for, not master of, practice). (Richardson et al 2004, p 203)

Knowledge and expertise

Schön (1988) contended that in order to deal with the crisis of professional knowledge and education, we need to recognise that outstanding practitioners do not have more professional knowledge but more wisdom, talent, intuition and artistry. Later Boshuizen and Schmidt (1992, 1995) developed a stage theory of the development of medical expertise, in which knowledge acquisition and clinical reasoning develop concurrently. This is essentially a theory of the acquisition and development of knowledge structures that provide the framework for clinical decision making. They contend that dramatic changes in clinical reasoning are the result of structural changes in knowledge. In this stage theory, the progression from medical student to expert clinician is accompanied by a transition from biomedical knowledge, through encapsulation of knowledge into concept clusters with clinically relevant foci to structuring of knowledge around *illness scripts* and, finally, to *instantiated scripts* (actual detailed cases or specific instances). This development in knowledge is accompanied by increasing expertise in reasoning. This model clearly identifies the importance of practice-generated, experiential knowledge.

In their grounded theory of expert practice in physical therapy, Jensen and colleagues (Jensen et al 2000, 2007, Shepard et al 1999) present expertise in physical therapy as a combination of multidimensional knowledge, clinical reasoning skills, skilled movement, and virtue, and contend that these four dimensions contribute to the practitioner's philosophy of practice. In this theory the experts' knowledge is multidimensional and patient-centred, and therapists draw from multiple sources including specialty knowledge and clinical knowledge gained through reflection on practice. Experts trust their craft or tacit knowledge and use it in making decisions about patient care. Again, experiential knowledge is vital alongside propositional knowledge.

Implications of ways of knowing for clinical education

Clinical education or professional development in the health professions occurs in a range of settings spanning acute care with seriously ill patients to longer term rehabilitation settings to non-clinical settings such as schools and industry. Common elements across these settings are a focus on health and/or healthcare, and the inherent ambiguities, unpredictabilities and complexities of any human services arena. Variations occur, as discussed above, in the model of education used and the model of practice promoted.

Conclusion

The chapter began with the argument that understanding of knowledge, its construction, context and use in practice is vital for good practice. It is also necessary for good learning and teaching in clinical education. In the last century one of the catchcries was the need for students to learn how to learn. In this chapter the challenge is that students and teachers need to know how to know. This can be done by explicit teaching and discussions about the nature and development of knowledge, by reflecting upon how novice and expert practitioners know and create knowledge in practice, and by examining practice experiences to study knowledge use in practice. For advanced practitioners, reflexive knowing or reflecting upon knowledge use and creation with subsequent development in knowing and knowledge base is an everyday but enriching way to enhance the capability for growth. For novices, the initial challenge is to know what is necessary and, at the same time, to identify what more can or should be known, including the art of knowing in practice.

- What difference does context make to knowledge use?
- How did your professional socialisation influence your views of knowledge and your ability to use knowledge generation and critique skills?
- What are desirable ways of learning or teaching about ways of knowing?

References

Aristotle 1985 Nichomachean ethics. trans. T Irwin. Hackett, Indianapolis (original c400 BC)

Bauman Z 2000 Liquid modernity. Polity Press, Cambridge

Bauman Z 2005 The liquid modern challenges to education. In: Robinson S, Katulushi C (eds) Values in higher education. Aureus, & the University of Leeds, Leeds, p 36–50

Berlin I (ed) 1979 Against the current: essays in the history of ideas. Hogarth Press, London

Boshuizen HPA, Schmidt HG 1992 On the role of biomedical knowledge in clinical reasoning by experts, intermediates and novices. Cognitive Science 16:153–184

Boshuizen HPA, Schmidt HG 1995 The development of clinical reasoning expertise. In: Higgs J, Jones M (eds) Clinical reasoning in the health professions. Butterworth-Heinemann, Oxford, p 24–32

Carper BA 1978 Fundamental patterns of knowing. Advances in Nursing Science 1:13–23

Cox A 2005 What are communities of practice? A comparative review of four seminal works. Journal of Information Science 31(6):527–540

Dibden M, Zakrzewski L, Hisggs J 2002 Australian occupational therapy: origins and directions. Focus on Health Professional Education: A Multi-Disciplinary Journal 4(3):1–20

Donovan J (ed) 1995 Health in Australia: what you should know. Australian Institute of Health & Welfare, Australian Government Publishing Service, Canberra

Eraut M 1994 Developing professional knowledge and competence. Falmer, London

Fish D, Coles C 1998 Developing professional judgement in health care: learning through the critical appreciation of practice. Butterworth-Heinemann, Oxford

Fish D, Higgs J 2008 The context for clinical decision making in the twenty-first century. In: Higgs J, Jones M, Loftus S, Christensen N (eds) Clinical reasoning in the health professions, 3rd edn. Elsevier, Edinburgh, p 19–30

Fulford KWM, Ersser S, Hope T (eds) 1996 Essential practice in patient-centred care. Blackwell Science, Oxford

Gustavsson B 2004 Revisiting the philosophical roots of practical knowledge. In: Higgs J, Richardson B, Abrandt Dahlgren M (eds) Developing practice knowledge for health professionals. Butterworth-Heinemann, Oxford, p 35–50

Higgs C, Neubauer D, Higgs J 1999 The changing health care context: globalisation and social ecology. In: Higgs J, Edwards H (eds) Educating beginning practitioners: challenges for health professional education. Butterworth-Heinemann, Oxford, p 30–37

Higgs J, Hunt A 1999 Redefining the beginning practitioner. Focus on Health Professional Education: A Multi-Disciplinary Journal 1(1):34–48

Higgs J, Titchen A 1995 Propositional, professional and personal knowledge in clinical reasoning. In: Higgs J, Jones M (eds) Clinical reasoning in the health professions. Butterworth-Heinemann, Oxford, p 126–146

Higgs J, Richardson B, Abrandt Dahlgren M 2004 Preface. In: Higgs J, Richardson B, Abrandt Dahlgren M (eds) Developing practice knowledge for health professionals. Butterworth-Heinemann, Oxford, p ix

Higgs J, Ajjawi R, Smith M 2008a Working and learning in communities of practice. In: Higgs J, Smith M, Webb G et al (eds) Contexts of physiotherapy practice. Elsevier Australia, Melbourne, p 117–127

Higgs J, Fish D, Rothwell R 2008b Knowledge generation and clinical reasoning in practice. In: Higgs J, Jones M, Loftus S, Christensen N (eds) Clinical reasoning in the health professions, 3rd edn. Elsevier, Edinburgh, p 163–172

Higgs J, Hummell J, Roe-Shaw M 2008c Becoming a member of a health profession: a journey of socialisation. In: Higgs J, Smith M, Webb G et al (eds) Contexts of physiotherapy practice. Elsevier Australia, Melbourne, p 58–71

Higgs J, Jones M, Titchen A 2008d Knowledge, reasoning and evidence for practice. In: Higgs J, Jones M, Loftus S, Christensen N (eds) Clinical reasoning in the health professions, 3rd edn. Elsevier, Edinburgh, p 151–161

James JE 1994 Health care, psychology, and the scientist–practitioner model. Australian Psychologist 29(1):5–11

Jensen GM, Gwyer J, Shepard KF et al 2000 Expert practice in physical therapy. Physical Therapy 80(1):28–43

Jensen GM, Gwyer J, Hack LM et al 2007 Expertise in physical therapy practice, 2nd edn. Saunders-Elsevier, St Louis

Kolb D 1984 Experiential learning: experience as the source of learning and development. Prentice-Hall, Englewood Cliffs, NJ

Larsen D, Loftus S, Higgs J 2008 Understanding knowledge as a sociocultural historical phenomenon. In: Higgs J, Jones M, Loftus S, Christensen N (eds) Clinical reasoning in the health professions, 3rd edn. Elsevier, Edinburgh, p 173–179

Lawson JS, Rotem A, Bates PW 1996 From clinician to manager: an introduction to hospital and health services management. McGraw-Hill, Sydney

Norman GR 1988 Problem-solving skills, solving problems and problem-based learning. Medical Education 22:279–286

Pynt J, Larsen D, Nicholls D et al 2008 Historical phases in physiotherapy. In: Higgs J, Smith M, Webb G et al (eds) Contexts of physiotherapy practice. Elsevier Australia, Melbourne, p 33–43

Richardson B, Abrandt Dahlgren M, Higgs J. 2004 Practice epistemology: implications for education, practice and research. In: Higgs J, Richardson B, Abrandt Dahlgren M (eds) Developing practice knowledge for health professionals. Butterworth-Heinemann, Oxford, p 201–220

Sahrmann SA 2002 Diagnosis and treatment of movement impairment syndromes. Mosby, St Louis, MO

Sarter B (ed) 1988 Paths to knowledge: innovative research methods for nursing. National League for Nursing, New York

Schön DA 1983 The reflective practitioner: how professionals think in action. Basic Books, New York

Schön DA 1988 From technical rationality to reflection-in-action. In: Dowie J, Elstein A (eds) Professional judgement. Cambridge University Press, Cambridge, UK

Sennett R 2005 The culture of the new capitalism. Yale University Press, New Haven

Shepard K, Hack L, Gwyer J et al 1999 Describing expert practice. Qualitative Health Research 9:746–758

Trede F, Haynes A 2008 Developing person-centred relationships with clients and families. In: Higgs J, Smith M, Webb G et al (eds) Contexts of physiotherapy practice. Elsevier Australia, Melbourne, p 246–249

Trede FV, Higgs J 2003 Reframing the clinician's role in collaborative clinical decision making: rethinking practice knowledge and the notion of clinician–patient relationships. Learning in Health and Social Care 2(2):66–73

Twomey L 1980 Making effective use of the physiotherapist. Patient Management 9(12):13–19

Twomey L 1990 A growing commitment to research and evaluation. Australian Journal of Physiotherapy 36(2):83

World Confederation for Physical Therapy 1999 Description of physical therapy. Declarations of principle and position statements approved at the 14th general meeting of WCPT, May 1999. Online. Available: http://www.wcpt.org/ Accessed 6 Jan 2009

World Health Organization 1986 The Ottawa charter for health promotion. Health Promotion 1(4):i–v

CHAPTER 3

Recognising and bridging gaps: theory, research and practice in clinical education

Sue Kilminster

THEORIES

Theories of cognitive psychology highlight that the context of learning and processes of participation are both highly influential in contributing to how a student 'recognises, acquires and organises' their knowledge. Sociocultural theories about learning focus on the situated nature of learning. This means the physical context, the type of participation and the development of relationships, all work to facilitate learning through a process of 'becoming' a member of the professional community and workplace.

USING THEORIES TO INFORM CURRICULUM DESIGN AND RESEARCH

When formulating goals of teaching there is a need to define the skills and competencies that the learner should acquire. In addition, it is important to acknowledge and include the nature and type of participation that is afforded to the student within the teaching scenario or experience.

USING THEORIES TO DRIVE EDUCATION METHODS

Example: When teaching a novice health practitioner a new clinical skill, it is important that the educator considers the assumptions they are making about their goals of teaching and their expectations of the learning process. Using theories about teaching and learning in the workplace or in clinical placement settings means that teaching strategies should be developed to foster students' engagement and integration into the practice community, in addition to structuring specific skill-based acquisition tasks.

Introduction

The purpose of this chapter is to examine the bases for contemporary theory, research and practice in clinical education and to consider how these might be informed and developed by a critique based on current understandings about learning. All understandings about clinical education in any healthcare profession, whether about its historical development, definitions, research or clinical education practices are underpinned by assumptions about learning. These assumptions determine the questions asked, the methods used to try to answer them, the conclusions drawn and the implications for clinical education practice and policies. However these assumptions are not usually made explicit in most of the relevant healthcare literature, nor indeed in that emanating from regulatory and professional bodies; consequently, the justifications for different theoretical approaches, research and practice remain under explored. Indeed many of the 'taken for granted' assumptions and ideas in contemporary clinical education research and practice are strongly contested in social science, particularly education, research and practice. This includes domination notions and conceptualisations about such issues as competence, generic skills, transfer, learning styles, attitudes, professionalism as well as the nature of much empirical work in clinical education.

Therefore, a key premise of this chapter is that understandings about learning must be made explicit and questioned in order to understand and develop theory, research and practice in clinical education. A second is that theory, research and practice are always interlinked, although this is not necessarily made explicit; ideas currently dominant in clinical education research and practice have the same theoretical and epistemological bases and each informs the other. These two premises underpin the arguments in, and structure of, this chapter, which begins with a consideration of some current conceptualisations and theoretical perspectives on learning in clinical settings. The second section deals with particular problems in clinical education research and the third section focuses on clinical education practice. The concluding section suggests some directions for development of theory, research and practice in clinical education.

I have developed the arguments in this chapter through my work in, and understanding of, medical education research, so it is specifically that research to which I refer most often. I have tried to indicate where my arguments are specific to medicine and where they are applicable to all healthcare professional education. My ideas have developed through collaboration with a number of colleagues, and I have drawn on some of our research for this chapter. In particular, I need to acknowledge working with Professor Miriam Zukas of the Lifelong Learning Institute at the University of Leeds on some of the ideas in this chapter.

Current conceptualisations and theoretical perspectives

It is difficult to define clinical education succinctly, certainly difficult to find a definition that everyone can accept, and even more difficult to reach consensus about its goals and purpose. There are many reasons for this but one of the most fundamental is epistemological; that is, to do with how knowledge and learning are conceptualised. Essentially clinical education is concerned with questions such as: What is the nature of clinical knowledge? How does an individual come to 'possess' it? How can they be helped in this process? How can we all know that a professional does 'possess' the requisite knowledge? Definitions of clinical education and statements about its goals and purposes contain implicit answers (or assumptions) to or about these questions. This section focuses on aspects of two theoretical perspectives, sociocultural and cognitive psychology, which I think can help us to both recognise and bridge some of the gaps in current research and practice in clinical education.

In most healthcare professional education research learning is usually investigated using individualistic psychological understandings and explanations of learning (Swanick 2005). That is, learning is understood as a process in which knowledge is somehow transmitted by the teacher and acquired by the learner. The research focus is usually on either the learner or the teacher, sometimes on the dyad, but generally little attention is paid to context. This is in contrast to much other education research that is predicated on sociocultural theories of learning in which learning is understood as a process of participation in activities which are situated in social and cultural contexts. Anna Sfard (1998) offered a useful analysis of understandings about learning by arguing that there are two current metaphors for learning—acquisition and participation—which guide learners, teachers and researchers. Learning, teaching and research are heavily influenced by whichever metaphor is used (often implicitly). She traces the acquisition metaphor back to Plato, while the participation metaphor has developed more recently in response to explanatory weaknesses in approaches that consider learning as a process of acquisition. Neither metaphor completely explains learning on its own, although it is clear that participation is a crucial but under used concept for clinical education.

Cognitive psychology perspectives on learning

Cognitive psychology research has demonstrated that by learning through participating in routine tasks and activities, concepts and activities are transformed into skilled performance that does not require conscious thought (compilation). Clinicians (and students) develop mental representations of cases—'illness scripts'—and their clinical reasoning appears to involve both analytical and non-analytical processes (Eva 2005) (see Ch 7). New learning and/or transfer is necessary to perform new and/or non-routine tasks and has been the subject of much debate (for example, Norman et al 2005, Colliver 2004). There is agreement that success in solving one clinical problem does not predict success at solving another, even related, problem and there is recognition that this is due to context specificity. However while this recognition has influenced current assessment practices, it seems to have had less impact on clinical education more generally. One of the main 'messages' of this chapter is that it is necessary to develop a much fuller understanding and recognition of contextual factors in order to develop more effective clinical education practices and research.

Sociocultural perspectives

Sociocultural perspectives understand learning to result from individuals constructing their own knowledge as a result of participating in sociocultural activity, for example, a healthcare student undertaking a clinical placement. Learning is situated (that is, contextual, dependent on the social and physical environment) and opportunities to participate—legitimate peripheral participation (Lave & Wenger 1991)—are therefore essential for learning. However these opportunities ('affordances') are dependent on many factors including hierarchies, acceptability, personal relationships and workplace culture, and so may not be equal (Billet 2001). Learning is usually understood as a form of internalisation in more individual psychological explanations but Rogoff (1995, Rogoff et al 1995) argues that change resulting from participating in an activity (which the authors call 'appropriation') is a process of transformation and not simply internalisation.

There are weaknesses in both perspectives. Cognitive psychology does not fully explain how knowledge is sourced, represented or constructed or how social practices influence this construction, while sociocultural theories do not completely account for the construction of different types of knowledge or how it is used (Billet 1998). So, in clinical education, cognitive psychology can account for aspects of the development of diagnostic skills, for example, but not how they are influenced by different settings and interactions. Conversely, sociocultural theories do not fully address how underpinning knowledge (and its 'accuracy' or otherwise) about bodily systems, for example, are used in activities although they do address how participation in activity influences learning. Both cognitive psychology and sociocultural perspectives understand (albeit with different emphases) knowledge acquisition as active and interpretative. Learning is understood more as a process of *becoming* in sociocultural theories, while in cognitive psychology perspectives it is more understood as a process of *making meaning*. Arguably, cognitive psychology privileges learning as a process of acquisition and sociocultural theories as a process of participation. Clearly how learning (and knowledge) is understood will determine both how it is investigated and how clinical education is delivered. I am trying to develop a research perspective that can explore and understand learning in clinical settings as involving both processes of becoming and making meaning.

Current empirical work

Research on clinical education encompasses assessment, clinical skills, communication skills, clinical teaching, supervision, community-based education, clinical reasoning, professionalism and many other topics. However, it is often either completely atheoretical or uses a concept (for example, learning styles, reflection, attitudes) without any justification of the use of that particular conceptual framework, underpinning assumptions are unquestioned and there is no acknowledgement of associated theoretical problems. Essentially much clinical education research is concerned with descriptive answers to the question 'What works?' Unless there is some understanding of how or why it 'works' such research is not helpful in developing deeper or more complex understanding about learning in clinical settings. Cook et al (2008) reviewed 105 studies describing medical 'education experiments' and found that 75 (72%) were justification studies (did it work?), 17 (16%) were descriptive (what was done), and only 13 (12%) were concerned with 'why or how did it work?' (clarification studies in their terminology). This review is particularly interesting because the authors are writing from within a scientific paradigm and have produced a similar critique to that developed from a more social sciences perspective. Both critiques centre on the problem that too many studies lack a theoretical framework and do not build on or address previous work (for example, Govaerts et al 2007, Kuper et al 2007, van der Vleuten & Schurwith 2005).

There is also a vast body of relevant social science research, particularly in education, that is largely ignored and often results in replication of research and/or debates that have already happened in other academic disciplines. However, I think that it can also be argued, at least to some extent, that other academic disciplines could benefit from considering aspects of clinical education research, but that would be a different chapter!

In this chapter I am going to consider some aspects of clinical education research with which I have been involved to illustrate these points in more detail.

Existing work in social sciences

There is a persistent trend in clinical education research to look for differences between groups, often without any consideration of the basis for, meaning or significance of postulating such differences. I will take the example of gender differences, although many of these arguments also apply to the search for differences between ethnic groups. It is rare that research papers considering gender differences make any acknowledgement of the longstanding, sophisticated and extensive debates and empirical work about gender and sex differences in the social sciences. One example will suffice to illustrate this point.

Janet Hyde (2005) examined 46 meta-analyses of research into gender differences in psychology. She found that 78% of reported gender differences were small or close to zero; the exceptions were throwing (particularly after puberty), and some measures of aspects of sexuality and physical aggression. However, in medicine, there are persistent ideas and research reports which suggest there are gender differences in motivations and attitudes, differences in academic performance, differences in clinical skills and communication skills, and even that women practice medicine differently. Our literature review (Kilminster et al 2007a) found very little evidence to support such arguments and assumptions; there is a vast amount of work that often produces conflicting findings. We did find problems with some of the research methodologies, frequent failure to report effect sizes, and, of course, there is also publication bias against non-significant findings.

It is essential to remember that '[h]ow we interpret data about the relative educational performance of different groups will depend on our research focus, and on our assumptions about the social and psychological processes involved' (Hammersley 2001, p 293). Furthermore, there is a strong argument that such research can be detrimental for women. Rosemary Pringle (1998) noted the trend in medical culture to exaggerate the 'feminine' qualities of women in communication, empathy and care; if women are considered to be good empathetic communicators this may confer short-term advantages over their male counterparts. However this may be a 'double-edged sword' that will ultimately restrict women to successful practice only as the 'new human face of a humbler form of medical practice'. Similarly, in the conclusion to her review of meta-analyses (2005) Janet Hyde argued that 'over inflated claims of gender differences … cause harm in numerous realms' (p 590) and, furthermore, such claims are also not consistent with the scientific data.

Research that aims to discern essential gender differences is often predicated upon unquestioned essentialist assumptions about traits and complementary skills that justify and reinforce women's subordinate position. Furthermore, the cultures and practices of all health professions are interrelated with the social contexts in which healthcare is delivered, so approaches aimed at isolating one factor, such as gender and communication skills, are likely to fail to identify, or explain, the complexities involved. In medicine, there is a lack of research and analysis into how male doctors are contributing to modern medicine that is indicative of the historically masculine context in which medicine is embedded—this is demonstrated by frequent reference to the 'feminisation' of medicine. It is female doctors who are researched as the 'other', whereas male doctors receive little attention. In the social sciences, gender is generally understood as a relation rather than a trait. Gender relations are maintained by the interaction of various processes at different levels; they are not fixed. Therefore future research will be best served not by assuming; or looking for sex differences, but by examining where gender becomes relevant and impacts on education, training, practice and career paths in healthcare.

Scientific approaches: the case of psychometrics

Clinical education research, especially in medicine, is often overly 'scientific'—concerned with 'objectivity' and accuracy—with insufficient recognition of the sociocultural context of clinical education and practice and the implications for research. This is particularly true of assessment. Assessment is a central concern in clinical education because ultimately clinical educators need to be sure that learners become able to deliver safe, appropriate and effective care. There is also a need, which is sometimes competing, to ensure that learners perceive assessment to be fair and to reassure the profession that it is accurate and 'objective'. These factors have led to the current emphasis on reliability, which is often confused with accuracy and notions of objectivity. Indeed, arguably, clinical educators practice defensive assessment.

Assessment research has been dominated by North American psychometricians, who have made significant contributions to the current practices of assessment. Indeed this approach provides the basis for the arguments of Chapter 9. However, as Kuper et al (2007) have recently pointed out, some aspects of practice 'are better thought of as social constructs. That is, instead of being considered as expressions of single individual's abilities, they are conceived of as the products of interactions between two or more individuals or groups' (p 1121). The ways in which people act are 'context-specific and culture-bound', therefore many of the attributes, abilities and competencies on which trainees are assessed are not fixed traits, nor do they exist independently of context as currently assumed. This has many implications for assessment practice. I will highlight only one of them: the use of standardised patients. These are people who are trained to portray specific clinical conditions or problems, and whose responses to the trainee are determined by a script that is intended to 'standardise' their interactions with different trainees. This can include prescribing dress, demeanour (including whether or not the patient becomes angry or upset), and other aspects that are actually context specific. This seems a completely illogical, indeed pointless, activity because no individual responds in the same way to different people—it is a case of over privileging reliability not reality (or validity). In contrast, simulated patients, who are also trained to portray specific clinical conditions or problems, offer a valid alternative because their responses are not predetermined but are determined by the nature of the interaction with the trainee or learner.

In the last few years there has been increasing attention on work-based assessments (Govaerts et al 2007, Schurwith & van der Vleuten 2006) although much work remains to be done to take more account of contextual factors, particularly in relation to working with others. For example, patient safety has been treated as if it were the responsibility of individuals but clinical practice is collegial and patient safety is the product of that collegiality (Lester & Tritter 2001).

Integrating research and theory: expertise

Theories about learning from experience and about the nature and development of professional expertise are highly relevant to understanding learning processes involved in clinical education. Generally theories of learning in medicine emphasise the importance of integrating experience, and make the point that learners are more able to deal with abstraction when they have more experience (Coles 1998). In order to become an expert practitioner, the trainee has to integrate knowledge gained from practice with pre-existing and/or theoretical knowledge. Much work on experiential learning (Kolb 1984, Boud et al 1993, Schön 1995) argues that reflection is central to this process—although there are, of course, very different understandings of reflection and reflective practice (Ch 1).

Expertise is difficult to define and can be hard to access because it involves tacit knowledge and skilled performance that often appears to become intuitive (Eraut 1994, 2004). Much of the empirical work concerned with the development of expertise in healthcare has examined diagnostic reasoning because it is a relatively discrete activity which can be subjected to experimental manipulation but still retain validity. The literature on expertise suggests that experts recognise patterns and meanings in information that are not noticed by novices; experts have extensive content knowledge, organised in 'deep' ways; context specificity is vital and experts appear to be able to retrieve knowledge with little effort; and experts may not be good teachers (Bransford & Schwartz 1999). Experts know what not to do in any situation while novice and intermediate practitioners do not (Patel & Groen 1991).

Empirical work shows that trainees expect more certainty about professional knowledge and practice than experts, partly because they appear to have different understandings of knowledge and partly because of their desire to avoid mistakes. For example, when specialist registrars were asked about their aims in supervision, they emphasised 'getting it right' and obtaining advice and reassurance (Cottrell et al 2002). Their emphases and reasoning were much more concrete than those of their supervisors who tended to describe broader more holistic aims. Pillay and McCrindle (2005) found that novices tended to rely on domain knowledge in diagnostic reasoning, while experts used more complex interactions; however the key to successful diagnosis was recognising important information, not complex reasoning. However, in clinical settings, trainees have to negotiate competing paradigms of certainty and uncertainty. Trainees have to learn to manage and live with uncertainty, while the discourse about evidence-based practice and adherence to treatment protocols suggests certainty about, and predictability in, practice outcomes. The cognitive psychology literature on expertise (Norman et al 2005) stresses the importance of context and practice, as well as knowledge, but it is still rooted in the asocial notion of expertise as something possessed by an individual and interactions are unexplored. Stephen Billett argues that we need a 'dynamic, negotiated and situated view of expertise' (2001, p 448) supplemented by a social and embodied understanding of knowledge and expertise. The relationships between these general issues and clinical education research and practice have yet to be developed. Indeed much current research shows more of the novice's search for certainty rather than the expert's tolerance for complexity and ambiguity.

Reconceptualising clinical education practice

I have argued that trainees' and trainers' understandings about learning affect how they construct both clinical practice and clinical education. This even affects what they see as learning; for example, a significant research finding is that clinical educators or supervisors identify more learning opportunities available to trainees than trainees recognise are available. There are a number of possible explanations for this. I think it is at least partly due to the separation between practice (or service delivery) and education and training. In previous work (for example, Kilminster & Zukas 2005, Kilminster et al 2007a), we have argued that the divide between clinical and educational supervision and between supervisory and facilitative functions of supervision is unworkable. Similarly, if learning is understood (even partly) from a sociocultural perspective as a process of becoming, then the divide between clinical practice and clinical education can be reformulated and a more complex workplace pedagogy developed. Currently clinical education tends to be based on a reductionist model in which separate skills are developed, but there is insufficient integration or structure—more recognition of the importance of context offers a route to developing clinical education pedagogy.

In this regard the literature on workplace learning offers some useful insights; perhaps most useful is the curriculum model suggested by Stephen Billett (2001). There are four elements in his suggested approach to workplace pedagogy:

1 movement from peripheral to full participation
2 access to goals for performance
3 direct guidance of experts and others
4 indirect guidance provided by the workplace.

Although Billett's model was developed for workplace learning more generally, all the above elements are relevant to clinical education, although the particularities of clinical settings do offer some challenges to his model. Billett argues that his structured approach to a workplace learning curriculum is technicist, cognitive, interpretivist and socially critical; that is, the approach encompasses learning which is instrumental in character; develops adaptable and robust (transferable) learning (p 136); acknowledges that learners are interpretative and selective in what and how they learn; and may facilitate socially critical understandings (such as about unequal opportunities, in workplaces, for access to practice)—all necessary attributes of clinical learning. It is useful to consider how far each of the above elements of a workplace curriculum can apply to learning in clinical settings.

Movement from peripheral to full participation

Lave and Wenger (1991) and many others since then have made the point that learning is ongoing practice, and that apprentices undergo (often systematically) a move from legitimate peripheral participation to full participation in any 'community of practice'. There is increasing recognition of the usefulness and potential of this way of understanding clinical education, but there are some problems with it. Particularly, there is a fluidity about clinical teams, which means that on some occasions a junior person might be the most senior present; for example, a junior doctor during an 'out of hours' emergency. In such situations normal hierarchical and power relations are disrupted for the sake of patient safety, and even the most junior trainees can have responsibilities which necessitate them acting as full participant, even though they are not. So in clinical education and training, the movement from legitimate peripheral participation to full participation is not always linear or systematic and changes due to contextual factors.

Access to goals for performance

Trainees' own goals and performance requirements are absolutely clear—to get the patient better! However these straightforward goals require a clinical team whose members may have differing goals and agendas. The complex professional arrangements and boundaries that surround the trainee may mean they have little understanding of the significance and detail of other professional groups' goals and actions. In this context other professional groups may have supervisory and other functions, but the existing context and dynamics could militate against them happening. For example, a junior doctor might be challenged by a pharmacist about a prescription, but if the junior doctor does not understand or accept the significance of the pharmacist's intention misunderstandings between the goals and intentions of the junior doctor and those of the pharmacist may create their own potentially life-threatening situation.

Direct guidance of experts and others

We (Kilminster et al 2007b) have shown empirically that direct guidance in medicine is far too infrequent and, even where guidance is given, there is little or no feedback. Feedback tends to be critical rather than constructive, and trainees may avoid seeking out such direct guidance as a result. Clinical settings present difficulties to structure direct guidance as Billett suggests. For example, one of the functions of direct guidance is to secure access to appropriate activities that should be sequenced from less to more complex, but this can be difficult in the context of service delivery where activities are dictated by patient needs, which can be very complex. A second function of direct guidance is to guard against inappropriate knowledge and practice; but a central problem with some clinical settings is that aspects of the knowledge and practice available to the trainee are inappropriate because of poor or outdated practices. Such conflicts between understandings and/or practices are very difficult for trainees.

Indirect guidance provided by the physical and social environment

That the workplace itself provides indirect guidance through the regular discussion and practice taking place in the clinical setting is very under recognised in clinical education, although this recognition could relieve some pressures on clinical educators if it were used appropriately. While there are many opportunities for indirect guidance and opportunities for learning are freely available, sometimes the indirect guidance available may also be inappropriate. For example, a number of studies have shown that undergraduate medical students' empathy is inversely related to their exposure to ward cultures and practices.

Summary

Our understanding about learning in clinical settings can be enhanced using sociocultural perspectives to develop a workplace curriculum such as that suggested by Billet. For example, the division between education and practice collapses when learning is recognised as an integral part of clinical activity. However, the focus on whole patients in complex service settings can challenge some of the assumptions behind workplace curriculum models. For example, individuals are positioned differently in relation to authority, responsibility and power depending on who else is present. Even a junior professional has a supervisory role at times. We need therefore to develop our understanding of clinical education practice in the light of the more fluid and multi-professional contexts in healthcare.

Future directions for research

I have argued that the underlying assumptions of both research and practice need to be made more explicit and to be questioned. Research needs to be informed by theoretical conceptualisations if we are to develop more sophisticated understandings about learning in clinical settings, and so develop clinical education practice. One important and helpful insight is that individual, social and cultural aspects of any activity are inseparable—although each can be a point of focus—and this therefore has implications for research on learning and development (Rogoff 1995, Rogoff et al 1995, Lave & Wenger 1991, Edwards 2005).

Sociocultural theorists (for example, Wertsch 1995, Engestrom 2001) contend that because an individual's actions cannot be separated from the social context, activity must therefore be the unit of analysis. 'Units of analysis focus on processes rather than on characteristics of individuals. Generalities are sought in terms of the nature of the processes as people participate in and constitute activities, rather than simply assuming context-free generality or seeking it in separated characteristics of the person or the task' (Rogoff et al 1995, p 126).

Rogoff (1995) identified three sociocultural planes in which work-learning occurs:

1 apprenticeship, which involves learning through engagement in community structures and activity

2 guided participation, the interpersonal process through which people are involved in sociocultural activity

3 participatory appropriation, how individuals change through their involvement in one or another activity.

These three planes are impossible to separate, except for the purpose of analysis, since one cannot exist without the others. Similarly, if more prosaically, the General Medical Council (GMC) in the United Kingdom identifies four levels of regulation: the individual, their clinical team (and the site where they are located), their employer, and the regulatory and policy context. Research and practice therefore need to account for all planes or levels. At first this seems to mean that research will become so complex that it will be extremely difficult to make any meaning or synthesis of research findings. However Hodkinson et al (2007) have suggested a useful metaphor: that of map making. In order to read a map it is necessary to understand its scale and to understand the information provided in relation and in context to that scale: this is true whether the map is small, medium or large scale. The information any map provides is only comprehensible if its scale is known. The same is true of research: the focus can be on a particular scale (or plane or level) but it has to be understood in context. The research has to take account of the different scales and to make clear how it is positioned in relation to them. Only then is it possible to identify the implications for practice and to understand how it is applicable to understanding about learning in clinical settings.

Conclusion

We need to use theory to explain, not to obfuscate or oversimplify, and to help understand learning in clinical settings. We need to attend more to levels of focus of research, questions addressed by it, and their significance and implications. How does it connect to other research and theory? What does it explain and why? Particular problems that need to be addressed by empirical work are to develop understandings about context and interactions. I am suggesting that we can recognise and bridge some of the gaps between theory, research and practice by conceptualising clinical education (research and practice) as a relational activity, not as a set of pedagogic practices carried out by one person upon another.

References

Billet S 1998 Appropriation and ontogeny: identifying compatibility between cognitive and sociocultural contributions to adult learning and development. International Journal of Lifelong Education 17(1):21–34

Billet S 2001 Learning in the workplace: strategies for effective practice. Allen & Unwin, Crows Nest, Sydney

Boud D, Cohen R, Walker D 1993 Using experience for learning. SRHE & Open University Press, Buckingham, UK

Bransford JD, Schwartz DL 1999 Rethinking Transfer: a simple proposal with multiple implications. Review of Research in Education 24:61–100

Coles C 1998 The educational supervisor's role in medicine. In: Peyton JWR (ed) Teaching and learning in medical practice. Manticore Europe, Rickmansworth

Colliver JA 2004 Full curriculum interventions and small-scale studies of transfer: implications for psychology type theory. Medical Education 38(12):1212–1214

Cook DA, Bordage G, Schmidt HG 2008 Description, justification and clarification: a framework for classifying the purposes of research in medical education. Medical Education 42(2):128–133

Cottrell D, Kilminster SM, Jolly B, Grant J 2002 What is effective supervision and how does it happen? Medical Education 36(11):1042–1049

Edwards A 2005 Let's get beyond community and practice: the many meanings of learning by participating. Curriculum Journal 16(1):49–65

Engestrom Y 2001 Expansive learning at work: toward an activity theoretical reconceptualisation. Journal of Education and Work 14(1):133–156

Eraut M 1994 Developing professional knowledge and competence. Falmer, London

Eraut M 2004 Informal learning in the workplace. Studies in Continuing Education 26(2):247–273

Eva K 2005 What every teacher needs to know about clinical reasoning. Medical Education 39(1):98–106

Govaerts MJB, van der Vleuten CPM, Schuwirth LWT, Muitjens AMM 2007 Broadening perspectives on clinical performance assessment: rethinking the nature of in-training assessment. Advances in Health Sciences Education 12(2):239–260

Hammersley M 2001 Interpreting achievement gaps: some comments on a dispute. British Journal of Educational Studies 49(3):285–298

Hodkinson P, Biesta G, James D 2007 Understanding learning cultures. Educational Review 59(4):415–427

Hyde JS 2005 The gender similarities hypothesis. American Psychologist 60(6):581–590

Kilminster S, Downes J, Gough B, Murdoch-Eaton D, Roberts TE 2007a Women in medicine: what's the problem? A literature review of culture and practice. Medical Education 41(1):39–49

Kilminster SM, Jolly BC, Grant J, Cottrell D 2007b Effective educational and clinical supervision. Medical Teacher 29(1)

Kilminster S, Zukas M 2005 Learning, life and death: theorising doctors' learning through the supervisory relationship. In: Boud D et al(eds) Researching work and learning conference. University of Technology, Sydney

Kolb DA 1984 Experiential learning experience as the source of learning and development. Prentice Hall, Eaglewood Cliffs

Kuper A, Reeves S, Albert M, Hodges BD 2007 Assessment: do we need to broaden our methodological horizons? Medical Education 41(12):1121–1123

Lester H, Tritter JQ 2001 Medical error: a discussion of the medical construction of error and suggestions for reforms of medical education to decrease error. Medical Education 35(9):855–861

Lave J, Wenger E 1991 Situated learning: legitimate peripheral participation. Cambridge University Press, UK

Norman GR, Eva KW, Schmidt HG 2005 Implications of psychology-type theories for full curriculum interventions. Medical Education 39(3):247–249

Patel V, Groen G 1990 The general and specific nature of medical expertise: a critical look. In: Ericsson KA, Smith J (eds) Towards a general theory of expertise: prospects and limits. Cambridge University Press, UK

Pillay H, McCrindle AR 2005 Distributed and relative nature of professional expertise. Studies in Continuing Education 27(1):67–88

Pringle R 1998 Sex and medicine: gender, power and authority in the medical profession. Cambridge University Press, UK

Rogoff B 1995 Observing sociocultural activity on three planes: participatory appropriation, guided participation and apprenticeship. In: Werstsch JV, del Rio P, Alvarez A (eds) Sociocultural studies of mind. Cambridge University Press, UK

Rogoff B, Radziszewska B, Maiello T 1995 Analysis of developmental processes in sociocultural activity. In: Martin L, Nelson K, Tobach E (eds) Cultural psychology and activity theory. Cambridge University Press, UK

Schön DA 1995 The reflective practitioner: how professionals think in action. Arena, Aldershot

Schuwirth LW, van der Vleuten CP 2006 Challenges for educationalists. British Medical Journal 333(7567):544–546

Sfard A 1998 On two metaphors for learning and the dangers of choosing just one. Educational Researcher 27(2):4–13

Swanick T 2005 Informal learning in postgraduate medical education: from cognitivism to 'culturalism'. Medical Education 39(8):859–865

van der Vleuten CPM, Schuwirth LWT 2005 Assessing professional competence: from methods to programmes. Medical Education 39(3):309–317

Wertsch JV 1995 The need for action in sociocultural research. In: Wertsch JV, del Rio P, Alvarez A (eds) Sociocultural studies of mind. Cambridge University Press, UK

Wertsch JV, del Rio P, Alvarez A (eds) 1995 Sociocultural studies of mind. Cambridge University Press, UK

Section 2

Sharing knowledge: communities and culture in education

CHAPTER 4

Professional identities and communities of practice

Gillian Webb, Rod Fawns and Rom Harré

THEORIES

Vygotsky's theory of cognitive psychology emphasises the importance of language and involvement in wider professional discourse as a means of facilitating learning. According to this theoretical perspective, for learning to be effective it must include an intention to share and understand the language, assumptions and aspirations of both the learner and the teacher.

Positioning Theory is an analytical framework that provides a way to view how people understand and interpret their rights and duties, or their 'position' in relation to another person. Using Positioning Theory facilitates analysis of the actions and language adopted by educators and students to aid understanding of, and insight into, the processes and effects of an education experience.

USING THEORIES TO INFORM EDUCATION PRACTICE AND RESEARCH

When formulating learning goals and teaching plans, it is important to attend to and include discourse about the learning event in addition to the skills required to be competent. Describing and discussing key features of a new skill or how to approach, assess or treat a particular patient provides a means to encourage both the learner and the teacher to explicitly acknowledge their positions and understanding, and most importantly to share their discursively based interpretation of a learning event.

USING THEORIES TO INFORM EDUCATION METHODS

Example: When teaching a novice health practitioner a new clinical skill, it is important to ensure there is an opportunity for a shared discussion about the new skill or ability. The shared discussion should encompass the educator's goals and expectations; the key learning objectives and the student's understanding and experience of the new learning event. Where relevant, the discussion should also encompass broader factors influencing the learning event based on the constraints and opportunities afforded by the particular clinical environment and people involved. To increase the effectiveness of learning in clinical education contexts, the expectations of learning and key educational outcomes should be discussed by both the educator and the learner.

Introduction

Clinical placements are fundamental to the educational experience of entry-level professionals. They are places where all students are inducted into the conversations of the health profession and begin to create their professional identity. Clinical placements, as a form of experiential learning, place demanding expectations on students. They are expected to demonstrate, often in unfamiliar situations, professional personae encompassing the application of technical knowledge and skill in site-specific contexts. Under direct supervision they are assessed for their ability to make responsible, safe and effective decisions about client welfare despite being at the intersection of various contingencies and necessities, initially only vaguely sensed (Webb 2004).

This chapter explores the idea that clinical placements and clinical practice for health professionals occur in communities of discourse. It seeks to illustrate a conceptual scheme that allows researchers, educators and students to follow the unfolding episodes of everyday life in clinical practices in new and illuminating ways. In this chapter we use two main theoretical frameworks as central anchors around which the importance of language and professional discourse are developed as mediums for clinical education learning. Our starting point is Vygotsky's (1962) conception of the person in an ocean of language, in intimate interaction with others, and in the flow of public and social cognition. From this discussion we move to the theoretical framework of Positioning Theory to provide a conceptual platform to underpin the dynamic nature of learning relationships within clinical healthcare settings.

Experiential learning

Experiential learning is not a new concept. Dewey (1933) wrote influentially about the relationship between experience and learning. His main thesis was that cognition is an interpersonal construct developed through language. Later writers, like Schön (1983, 1987) have drawn on Dewey's work to ground professional learning in rational reflection on one's practices. Discussions about the nature of different forms of knowledge suggest truth and knowledge may be revealed in the practical consequences of an action or investigation (Gustavsson 2004). In this chapter, our central theme is that clinical practice and learning professional skills in clinical placement settings is a social act and not simply learning a professional role as a bundle of behaviours—like reading an instrument accurately. In proposing this argument, we rely on authors such as Vygotsky (1962), Wittgenstein (1953), Harré & van Langenhove (1999) and others, who have argued that mental life presupposes the giving of and asking for reasons for what we think, feel and value. This means, in a practical sense, that a novice's actions are indissoluble from their speech and constituted in communities of practice in normative rather than causal connections.

According to Vygotsky, the sources of higher order cognitive processes like remembering, reasoning and classifying are socially rather than cognitively based. His principles of learning are grounded in psychological theory and underpin our key contention that learning in clinical placements should be recognised as a social and discursive activity.

Application of Vygotsky's principles to clinical education

Vygotsky (1962) placed great emphasis on the role of language, not just as an attribute of individuals, but rather as the medium of interpersonal conversations. In these conversations, cognitive problems are solved and cognitive tasks performed. By appropriating or 'taking on' the discursive means in a community of practice, the individual becomes a competent individual performer. By appropriation we are suggesting that the routine nature of professional practice and knowledge needs to be integrated with the reflective and emerging thoughts of the novice, to ensure that there is a level of consistency and understanding between the thoughts and language of the novice and those of their peers.

In new clinical contexts, novices' actions lack coherence in the local professional culture to whose membership they aspire. According to Vygotsky (1962), language and thought are two streams, one social and the other individual, which flow together in the higher cognitive functions, such as reasoning, deciding and remembering. Vygotsky introduced the idea of the acquisition not only of material tools but of cognitive tools, symbolic systems of which the most important was language. Vygotsky's view is that language is the mediating tool of all higher order cognitive functions, and it is in the conversations in the family circle and among one's peers that psychological development occurs.

The key to Vygotsky's psychology is the idea of a kind of 'psychological symbiosis' where the senior member in a relationship scaffolds the learning of the junior member. Vygotsky (1962) proposed that every cognitive function is a joint project between the senior member and the junior member, where the junior member appropriates the new knowledge as their own. Although Vygostsky's model was traditionally applied to childhood cognitive psychology, it can be extrapolated to adult learning situations. Understanding the learning process in symbiotic relationships is highly relevant to the learning that occurs in clinical placements. For example, when a novice is confronted by a task beyond their capabilities, they may try to perform the task but fail. Close by is the clinical educator, more able. The clinical educator, realising what the novice is trying to do, fills in the missing moves needed to complete the task successfully. The novice copies the supplementary moves next time they are confronted with a similar task. At the beginning of this process, the task and the novice's capabilities are what Vygotzky calls the 'zone of proximal development' (ZPD).

There is a direct link here to clinical education pedagogy. Inter-psychological functioning between student and educator must be structured so as to enhance the development of intra-psychological functioning in the student. Feedback conversations form a prime example of this inter-psychological functioning between student and educator. In clinical practice the student demonstrates their skills and explicates their thinking, and the clinical educator evaluates these practices in relation to norms of practice through the provision of feedback. There is an expectation that the student will, in turn, appropriate this new information produced in feedback conversation, and that the transformation will be evidenced in their future practice. 'Instruction in the zone of proximal development "calls to life in the (novice), awakens and puts in motion an entire series of internal processes of development".' (Vygotsky 1962, p 71)

Learning through engagement: professional or personal practice knowledge

Vygotsky's theories of psychology and their influence on the psychology of learning suggest that professional knowledge should not be reduced to practical or technical-based knowledge, but should incorporate the learner's own experiences and interpretations. Eraut (1985) and Williams (1998) discussed professional knowledge as having three components. The first is propositional knowledge, derived from discipline-based theories and concepts or from bodies of systematic knowledge that are publicly available. The second is personal, tacit or dispositional knowledge acquired by experience, and the third is process knowledge consisting of knowing how to conduct the various processes that contribute to professional accomplishment, including how to access and make use of propositional knowledge. Based on these distinctions, they described professional knowledge as the holistic integration of propositional, personal and process knowledge. Indeed on the basis of the layered nature of professional knowledge, one might argue that it needs to be rescued for the novice from assumptions of a routine nature.

In the development of clinical knowledge for novices, both the social and physical environments mediated by a preceptor–educator provide important contexts for learning. However the personal context (that is, the novices' views of themselves) are also highly significant. Clandinin & Connelly (1987) described this personal context as 'personal practical knowledge'. In order to develop, it requires both private and public reflective thought in and about practice, and not just a process of direct transmission of information from a mentor. Figure 4.1 illustrates this concept of teaching–learning that we are promoting in this chapter.

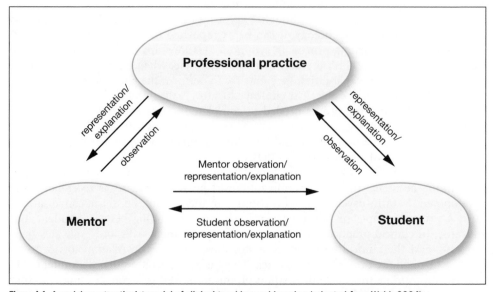

Figure 4.1 A social constructionist model of clinical teaching and learning (adapted from Webb 2004)

Pickering (1990) is another author who, like the more theoretically based Vygotsky, discussed the nature of the interpersonal relationship between students and educators as important to learning. She suggested that learning that occurs through relationships draws on cognitive knowledge; knowledge gained through prior experience and as an outcome of reflection on that experience through personal action. From this basis, enactment or practical experience should ideally provide the context for the development of understanding of competing perspectives. These perspectives include the proper technical management of a patient's condition and clarification of how normatively based or discipline specific and rule-based reasoning relates to individual client needs.

Reason and Heron (1986) observed that professional experience enables knowledge to be gained through encounters with others, through a practising of skills as one engages in professional activities and associated reading and reflection. The encounters may be direct, as in being given direction or observation, or they may be indirect, such as through conversation. But in all cases they are mediated by previous knowledge and the intentions of the persons involved. They most often contain an affective element indicative of being in relationship. Bateson (1979) similarly argued that clinical learning is a holistic process that has affective, cognitive and conative features.

The following quotes are derived from the work of Webb (2004) whose research explored how physiotherapy students develop professional identity through conversations with others. The data illustrate the integral nature of students' personal frames of reference and thoughts on their learning experience and outcomes. In the quotes, pronouns are bolded as a means of highlighting personal agency (Muhlhausler & Harre 1990).

In the quotation below, the student's comment reflects the interpersonal signing that is fundamental to experiential learning; that is, the accepting and valuing of himself, which enabled him to go on with his learning.

> Well, initially **I** sort of treated **her** like as a supervisor and **I** was like a student type thing, **I** think **I** was waiting there for **her** to give me some information at first and that's why **I** think **I** didn't go very well at the beginning … later on **we** didn't concentrate on just **my** learning then because **we** started, more towards sort of like a colleague type relationship afterwards, because **I** was actually progressing and **she** was happy and **she** was confident in me and **I** was confident. (Webb 2004, p 114)

In this next quotation, the student indicates an aspiration to join a community of practice with its norms and rules.

> Well in the clinics **I** hope to be able to interact more, like observe other clinicians. And sort of learn from their behaviour and learn from their actions. Just like as to know what is right and what is wrong and what's appropriate and what's not appropriate at certain times. (Webb 2004, p 26)

The two quotations above illustrate through students' eyes a motivation to learn through engagement and dialogue. In the next section, the importance of students' motivations, expectations and ways of identifying themselves are highlighted to further illustrate the influence of intra-psychological functioning on the nature and processes of learning.

Student expectations

Students have their own expectations of clinical practice. For example, they expect in their placements to make the transition from an isolated to a collegial existence. They expect to be accepted as a person, to get on well with significant others in the clinical situation, to be helped to perform well, to pass any assessments and make a recognised contribution. They expect to successfully put into practice what they feel they already know, in addition to learning new aspects of practice. Many emotions come with these expectations of self and of others. As Schatzki (2003) observes, in clinical practice placements, students expect their professionalism to be born, to unfold and to develop.

Some important implications of these expectations are that students rely on their prior academic studies to have taught them the authentic scientific *language* required in clinical practice. This will allow them to be able to communicate effectively and authoritatively with clinical educators, patients, their families and other professional colleagues, and to be recognised for these skills. However the *language of practice* is new to many students and has its own implicit local rules and cultural uses that need to be learnt. Webb (2004) found the process of mastering this implicit knowledge is complex for most students, particularly when communicated in a second language and culture. Crucial moments in becoming a professional are often couched in successful or unsuccessful moments in conversational interactions that are not limited to words in clinical settings.

Learning and professional identity formation is strongly influenced by the psychological positioning, institutional practices and societal rhetoric of the local discourse community. The ability of the individual student to locate themselves within these social episodes is complex and requires an understanding of both the explicit and the implicit rules and practices (Webb 2004). These implicit rules or norms are often embodied in 'second nature' practices grounded in local cultural assumptions that are rarely scrutinised.

The claims discussed previously by Vygotsky and others are that if local cultural assumptions and professional identity are not carefully scrutinised or made explicit and combined with students' expectations arising from their own cultural assumptions and learning expectations, then the learning process may be less effective. The cultural psychologist Ratner (2000) also endorses these claims through his criticism of the dominant individualistic view of cultural agency that often frames professional education in universities. He claims that Western university courses implicitly teach 'individual agency' and that individual acts are considered to be the most significant in the learning process. Related to this view of learning and contribution to a societal group is the idea that individual constructions of personal meaning are more creative and profound and that personal-social virtues, such as 'adaptability' or 'perceptiveness', are often viewed as individual constructions.

Through this critique, Ratner contends that the main problem with an individualistic view of cultural agency is that it may 'silence' clinical conversations of those students who do not share the dominant culture (p 414). Ratner (2000, p 415) also observes that 'institutional practices are not simply suggestions or meanings that can be ignored with impunity. Institutions are entities which structure people's psychology by imposing rules of behaviours, punishments, rewards etc. They are controlled by a group of people and are not negotiated by individuals'. Ewing and Smith (2001, p 16) argue further that the novice's aspiration for community membership is also bound to their biographies, their own storylines about 'doing, knowing, being and becoming'. Practice is about self-improvement with and for other people within a purposeful informed ethical and aesthetic framework. These views support the importance of the central theme of this chapter, that student learning cannot effectively take place from a position of passive transmission of views from an educator to a student. There needs to be a recognition and active steps taken to integrate the personal, the cultural and the institutional.

Novices expect to be able to transform their theoretical knowledge into explicit practice knowledge. They expect opportunities to discuss with others their emergent personal knowledge in critical areas of practice, to have their position supported or refuted. They expect community recognition from, as well as accountability to, significant others. From these expectations, interpersonal relations provide a means of entering into communal forms of remembering, deciding and problem solving.

Among the most important types of communal obligations are rights and duties and their distribution in the clinical community. Students expect to participate in this local moral order; that is, to fully explore their rights and duties in the clinical community. Through this need for a more engaged style of learning, we argue that the evolution of the profession and the transformation of organisational capacity in clinical communities depend on how well students understand their own agency in this dual praxis of exercised rights and duties. This understanding is influenced by the opportunities they are given to join or integrate with the professional community. This theme is developed further here and is elaborated in Chapter 7 in the evolution of professional reasoning.

Learning through enculturation and personal professional identity formation

Wenger (1998) highlights five cultural dimensions of personal professional identity that we also discuss in this chapter:

> Identity as negotiated experiences where we define who we are by the ways we experience our selves through participation as well as the way we and others reify ourselves: Identity as community membership where we define who we are by the familiar and the unfamiliar: Identity as learning trajectory where we define who we are by where we have been and where we are going: Identity as nexus of multi membership where we define who we are by the ways we reconcile our various forms of identity into one identity: Identity as a relation between the local and the global where we define who we are by negotiating local ways of belonging to broader constellations and manifesting broader styles and discourses. (Wenger, p 149)

We recognise that both novices and their mentors will not always be able to articulate these identities and positions, or have well-defined reasons for what they do. Faced with many contingencies, in most critical situations we do not have conscious aims and corresponding justifications. Social agents engaged in front-line clinical management will not always have reasons to act, or have reasons that direct, guide or orient their actions. Indeed they may engage in reasonable forms of behaviour without, for example, rationally following predetermined treatments.

We are arguing that a professional's public and private psychological life depends on discursive practices of giving and receiving reasons for actions—often retrospectively constructed. Moreover, we contend that without such language-related development, personal identity formation and social representations that embody collective identity may not be well formed. When Aristotle defined the human animal as a rational animal, he did not mean that we always act rationally but referred rather to our capacity for conceptual thinking and speech, our capacity for argument, and for responding to reasons and rationales for clinical decisions. This capacity in the novice or mentor will not always be exercised explicitly on a moment-by-moment basis. In the clinical placement setting, we locate reasons for action in the practices that constitute the mental life of the clinical setting, rather than in some private mental realm where it is commonly thought to reside. Schein (1978) framed professional identity as a longitudinal construct, developed through varied experiences and feedback that allowed the student to self-regulate their practice.

Webb (2004) found students' self efficacy to learn was challenged if their ethnic identity, and in particular their English language competence, was viewed as a barrier to entry to the psychological location in the local moral order of the clinic. She found that when the student or preceptor does not participate in the public mental life of the community of practice, the processes of professional identity formation are likely to remain obscure if not closed to the student.

In the quote below, the student forcefully positions himself positively in relation to the local moral order.

> I guess it's important to establish what kind of person **you** are and definitely why **you** are in this clinic. So I guess I should establish that I'm here to learn not because it's only part of the curriculum to get a pass, but I'm here actually to experience what it's supposed to be like in the actual workplace. And to probably, umm, to project a professional image, not so much as a student, but as a budding professional. (Webb 2000, p 144)

The student in the extended quote below reflects on the social–psychological processes we call 'appropriation', 'internalisation' and 'publication' that are involved in professional identity formation in different clinical settings. The quote demonstrates that the private–public interactions are not always linear or unidirectional in time.

> I began to be more reflective to suggestions from colleagues, fellow physios and supervisors. I tried to cultivate an expression of openness to **my** supervisors by providing a logical reasoning behind **my** actions, but as I find later too much information can be a hindrance as well. Being perceived as being defensive, I was struggling to alter that perception. In the end, I was being defensive about **me** being defensive, which in retrospection yields an amusing chuckle or two. I guess the way in which I communicated with **my** supervisor changed from too much information at the beginning of each block to insufficient information, as I felt worn out and resigned to whatever suggestions were given.

> As much as I see **myself** as an equal of the supervisor as a person (this does not mean that I see **myself** as of the same experience, but somebody who deserves respect), I cannot help but perceive a power difference that I felt was blatantly displayed at times during feedback sessions. I must admit that on the whole, supervisors have patience aplenty to accommodate **my** ramblings. In the end, I find it hard to position **myself** as somebody with a right to voice **my** opinion, it slowly developed into a more rigid team leader/ member hierarchy, similar to that found in corporate offices. Geelong was different in this respect, as I find a casualness amongst physios which I was comfortable with. Overall though, it was like 'do this **my** way, and say something only if it was worthwhile'. Which makes sense in a system running on the edge, and it is only human nature to expect one's pupils to follow the way the one prefers. (Webb 2004, p 159)

When students are required to conform to an unreflective process of professionalisation, they will often comment on the need to 'play the game' in the clinical context. They see their supervisor–mentor holding considerable power over their admission to the profession, and say it is wiser to appear to accept their mentor's position than to venture their own position in public discourse. To avoid this exclusionary and potentially damaging learning environment, it is important to be aware of and to actively use the positive force of a professional 'culture' and community of practice. This means students should be encouraged in their clinical experiences to develop realistic views of the challenges, as well as the opportunities, that are available for self cultivation in the local and wider cultural context of these experiences. This involves having a view of a professional community and the culture of that community as a dynamic structure.

Culture is the medium through which people's understanding of work practices, attitudes and behaviours are learned and shaped (Wolcott 1988). The culture of a professional community of practice is also the medium through which identity and practice are intimately connected to address social and political purposes. This means that learning is closely associated with the context in which it is learned. Moreover the intensity of the interaction between the public and private domains will continue to influence the development of their normative reasoning with the potential to affect their professional learning and their professional identity formation. The focus in the next section is on the private domain of identity formation, including theories that provide a platform for understanding and negotiating identity formation over time.

Temporality and self identity

How do students participate in their own identity formation over time? Not only do the tools of thought and action change with time, but so too do the distributions of rights and duties among a group of people who work together over short and longer periods. The individuals involved in communal cognitive activities over time are the bearers of a complex and labile psychology, some of which can be captured in a discussion of 'selves'. The English word 'self' does not translate easily into most other languages, but the concept can be appropriated as a technical term for our purposes here. We must take account of how the mutability and multiplicity of self ties in rights and duties in thought and action.

Persons 'have' selves. Three main items in personhood that the word is currently used to identify include first, the *embodied self,* which comes down to the unity and continuity of a person's point of view and of action in the material world, a trajectory in space and time. The embodied self is singular, continuous and self-identical. Then there is the *autobiographical self,* the hero or heroine of all kinds of stories. Research has shown how widely the autobiographical selves of real people can differ from story to story. Then there is the *social self* or selves, the personal qualities that a person displays in their encounters with others. This 'self' too is multiple. Psychologists use the phrase 'self-concept' to refer to the beliefs that people have about themselves, their skills, their moral qualities, their fears and their life courses (Harré & Moghaddam 2003).

What can change? Clearly the embodied self is invariant under the kind of transformations that occur in everyday life. Changing jobs or partners, the birth and death of family members, even moving into a new linguistic community, does not disrupt the continuity of the trajectory of life through space and time. When memories fade and anticipation of the future dims, the continuity of self fades with it and, though a living human body is before us, sometimes we are forced to acknowledge it is no longer an embodied self. However the repertoire of social selves and the stories with which one marshals one's life may and do change, sometimes in radical ways.

Persons have rights and duties, which are also distributed in a variety of ways depending on many factors, some of which involve the selves comprising the personhood of an individual. Here we encounter the province of 'Positioning Theory', the study of the way rights and duties are taken up and laid down, ascribed and appropriated, refused and defended in the fine grain of the encounters of daily lives in clinical and other social episodes.

Positioning Theory

Shared assumptions about local systems of rights and duties influence small-scale interactions in everyday conversations in clinical settings. 'Positioning Theory' framed by Davies and Harré (1991) is an analytical tool useful in the study of changes in local systems of rights and duties. The nature, formation, influence and ways of change in systems of rights and duties are all encompassed.

A 'position' is a metaphorical location taken in the psychological space afforded a person in a particular social episode or clinical conversation, whereby any participant may publicly claim more or less right, responsibility or duty to act. Any particular conversation affords only certain positioning opportunities for speakers to locate or relocate themselves in the local moral order. Each person can position themselves deliberately or adopt a position in response to the expectations of others in the conversation or outside it. They may position themselves with or without conscious intent.

Positioning Theory is to be seen in contrast to the older framework of Role Theory. Roles as bundles of behaviours are relatively fixed, often formally defined and long lasting. The person themself tends to be ignored in role descriptions. Even such phenomena as 'role distance' and 'role strain' presuppose the stability of the roles to which they are related. Positioning Theory concerns conventions of speech and action used by persons as accounts of their agency: they are labile, contestable and ephemeral.

To appreciate the significance of positioning analyses, it is important to reflect on some main features of the relations between language and thought, and language and action. Thinking has many forms, but the form that is of paramount importance for most people is thinking as the use of cognitive tools to carry out the tasks of everyday life. The most important cognitive tools are symbols, usually words and other language-like devices, and models and other forms of iconic representation. As we have already indicated, only relatively recently has it been realised by psychologists that thinking can be communal as well as individual, public as well as private. This has particular significance in research and practice in clinical education where learning and instruction occur in practice communities, and the distinctiveness of the everyday discourses to which students aspire to be inducted.

We have argued in this chapter that language is the prime instrument of thought and social action in professional education. This contention is made against the presupposition of much psychological research, namely the stability and transpersonal intelligibility (or transparency of meaning between people) of language. In so far as there are psychologically significant varieties of language and uses of language in the clinical setting, among the clinical educators, students and patients, so there are other dimensions of multiplicity of selves in the clinical setting.

This insight leads to reflections on the question of where and when people are thinking in a certain way in a social episode. The domain of thinking is intrapersonal and interpersonal. Thinking is not only an individual–personal activity but also a social–public one. For example, the process of remembering includes conversational as well as introspective activities. Students among themselves, with their university tutor or clinical educator discussing a particular interesting case, each contribute something to the construction of a version of the treatment and its effect. It is communally constructed, and each member takes away with them some version of that version on which further action is often based. It follows that there are exterograms, records of the past outside the brain of a person, as well as engrams, traces of the past incorporated in the long-term memory. There are legible material things, such as treatment notes, professional reports, and patient claims. There are the relevant sayings and doings of other people. These are all resources for acts of remembering, often overriding personal recollections.

There are plenty of examples of thinking spanning both the individual–personal and social–public domains. In deciding what to do, a student will spend time on private reflections of the consequences of a plan of action, perhaps attempting to imagine the future in some concrete way. However often there are public discussions, people go about seeking advice on the best course of action. There are influences from the unstated opinions of others, which may show up indirectly in what they do and say. There are informal varieties of the formal decision procedures involving problems, procedures, priorities, agendas, resolutions, amendments, and so on.

From whence comes the content of the beliefs with which positioning acts are supported and/or engendered? The way positioning acts work depends on two clusters of beliefs. The most basic are the beliefs people have about the character of the rights, duties and obligations that are constitutive of the local moral order. Allied with and supporting many of the actual positioning acts that people engage in are also beliefs about the way that personal characteristics, practical, intellectual, moral and characterological support or undercut positionings, whether it be by self for self or by others to self. The answer according to the Vygotskian account of human development must be found in the many patterns of psychological symbiosis by which not only the form of consciousness is formed but also a good deal of the content that emerges in such practices as positionings.

Clearly in a vibrant discursive community of clinical practice, interpersonal relations enter into communal forms of remembering, deciding, and problem solving. Among the most important are rights and duties and their distribution among the people involved. But our central argument for the importance of everyday workplace conversation in shaping personal identity formation and organisational renewal is not grounded only in interpersonal communication. Our interest in conversation as the basic social entity encompasses meanings in all semiotic interactions, speech, gestures and practices.

Conditions of meaningfulness

There are three relevant background conditions for the meaningfulness of a flow of symbolic interactions. The media of such interactions include linguistic performances, but also other symbolic systems. People make use of patient requests, professional standards, accredited procedures, rostered duties, workplace agreements, conditions, rights and duties, clinical data bases, authority figures and so on in the maintenance of the flow of actions constitutive of a clinical social episode.

a The first background determinant of meaning among participants in a conversation is the local repertoire of admissible social acts and meanings, in particular the illocutionary (strategic) force of what is said and done. Illocutionary force is the effective, then and there social significance, of what is said or done (Austin 1959). The same verbal expression or gesture may have a variety of meanings depending on who is using it, where and for what. Uttering 'I'm sorry', for instance, may in certain circumstances be the performance of an apology. It may also, in the United Kingdom, be a way of asking someone to repeat what has just been said. It may be a way of expressing incredulity.

b The second condition is the implicit pattern of the distribution of rights and duties to make use of items from the local repertoires of the illocutionary forces of various signs and utterances. Each distribution is a position. A professional has the right to assert, 'We don't do it that way here', but a novice or visitor does not. Professionals have a duty to attend meetings while novices and visitors do not. Positions have this in common with roles, that they pre-exist the people who occupy them, as part of the common knowledge of a community, family, sports team and so on. Both are psychological locations but also have a skill dimension. A professional head may have the moral authority by virtue of their title or office to distribute rights and duties in the community of practice but lack the moral capacity or skill to effect changes to conventions of practice.

c Third, every episode of human interaction is shaped by one or more story-lines which are usually taken for granted by those taking part in the episode, such as the shared assumptions about the clinic's charter, the role of the patient in their own treatment and the confidentiality of personal information. There are strong connections also to autobiographical psychology, the study of how, why and when people 'tell their lives' and to whom. A problematic client interaction may be told as a 'heroic quest', and what would have been complaints about overservicing according to one story-line become bureaucratic or accounting obstacles bravely overcome to meet basic patient needs. A solicitous remark to a novice can be construed as caring according to one story-line, but as an act of condescension according to another (Davies & Harré 1990).

These three basic background conditions in conversation, admissible acts, positioning and story-lines, comprise a mutually determinant triad, represented schematically in the positioning triangle (Fig 4.2), that structures the moment-by-moment meaning-making in professional discourse and action in and about institutional practices, positioning and societal rhetoric in clinical settings.

The positioning 'triangle'

Challenges to the way a clinical episode is unfolding can be directed to any one of the three conditions by any participant. We can represent this mutuality schematically as follows.

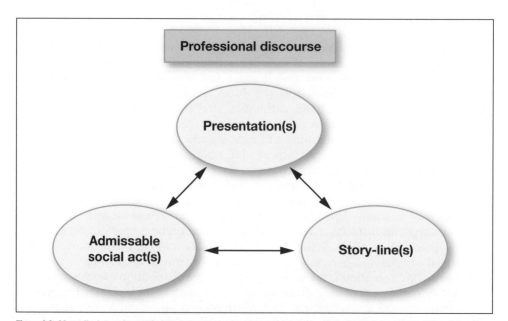

Figure 4.2 Mutually determinate triad that structures meaning-making in the flow of action in communities of practice

Each such triangle is accompanied by shadowy alternatives into which it can modulate or which can sometimes exist as competing and simultaneous readings of events by participants. In the socialisation of newcomers to the profession, they must not only acquire new skills but also adopt the social norms and rules that govern how they must conduct themselves. These are often implicit and not made obvious to newcomers. Professional identity formation will typically occur in the flow of action between the preceptor–educator and the student as they attempt to make determinate the implicit meanings in their interactions in each social episode (Richardson 1999).

It is important therefore that professional learning fosters a familiarity and confidence in discursive practice, which will increase the ability of students to present and pursue their ideas. The identity formation process may be described as a spiral, where a dynamic and dialectic equilibrium is maintained between the formation and maintenance of structure (that is, commitment and definition of self, 'where do I position myself?', 'how am I expected to act?') and flexibility and openness to change (that is, exploration, 'dare I try this?'). Early clinical experiences are particularly contradictory and ambiguous, stimulating fundamental self-reflection and questioning of one's personal views. Earlier ways of thinking and doing appear no longer appropriate in the situation at hand, and the individual is faced with the need to consider alternative resolutions and views. Niemi (1997) reminds us that when we try to communicate commitments, we enter the public realm and are more likely to become more conscious of our own implicit way of thinking in response to social expectations or needs. At the intersection of these needs and our own purposes, we frame the rules for our professional behaviour and maybe others. In the process of transforming ourselves in conversation, we may thus transform the institution. These mutually determining aspects of identity formation and institutional reform are shown in schematic form in Figure 4.3. They include processes of sharing ideas and knowledge (publication); learning through observation of others (conventionalisation); beginning to absorb professional goals by setting own goals within a professional discourse (transformation); and then constructing and testing personal understanding and interpretation of professional learning (appropriation).

Professional knowledge, as we have indicated, is constructed by health professionals through the three-way integration of procedural and propositional knowledge with experiential knowledge, which is mainly tacit and individual (Polanyi 1969). Participation with important others (Vygotsky 1962) towards an appreciation of the contextual detail of healthcare events provides the guidance or scaffolding relevant to the achievement of good healthcare practice in changing contexts. Professional identity formation can be viewed as a process of self-cultivation and development of professional agency, which concentrates on the student's struggle to achieve more enhanced levels of self-realisation.

A transformational model of clinical education: generating a community of practice

We propose a transformational model of clinical education as a summary of our position discussed in this chapter (Fig 4.4). The model situates clinical education as a social constructivist activity in which the manner in which humans make sense of their world is through everyday discourse, freely developing personal constructs that they test continuously in their community of practice, leading to transformation of that community of practice. Webb (2004) and Phillips et al (2002) identify in different health education

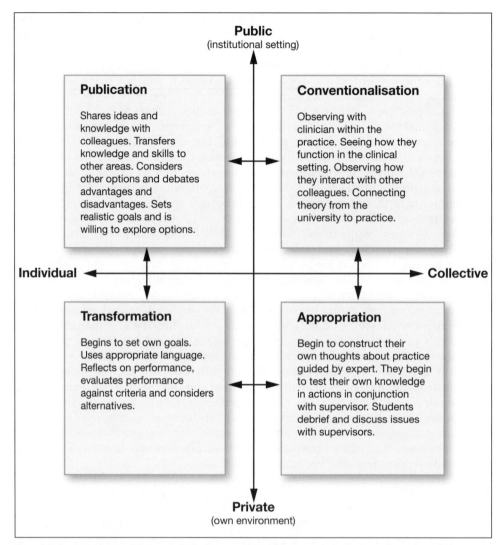

Figure 4.3 A representation of the psychological space within which personal identity formation occurs within a social episode (Webb 2004)

practices how Positioning Theory can be used to analyse the underlying structure of presuppositions that influence the unfolding of a teaching and learning episode. Students bring their own biographies and story-lines to the tasks of the community. The story-lines will normally be about their employment or the possible employment of accessible resources that often come to define the rules of practice. In a community of discursive practice, members in any social event or conversation will be repositioning themselves and/or others. From these theoretical claims, clinical learning can be seen as a type of repositioning. If there is little repositioning and it 'all seems very familiar', then, we suggest, there may also be little possibility of learning. Where a novice encounters a 'completely new world', major repositioning may be required.

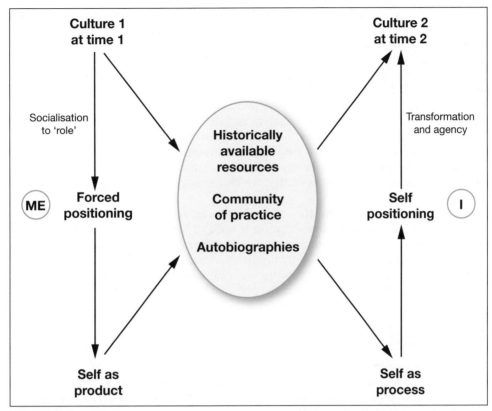

Figure 4.4 Model of transformation of personal identity and the profession of physiotherapy (Webb 2004 adapted from Bhaksar 1993)

The transformational model of social action presented in Figure 4.4 locates actual transformation of the profession in a dualism of praxis between agency and structure (self as product and self as process). Culture 1 in the figure represents the social structures manifest in the rules and resources of practice and rhetoric that determine the structures through which students are socialised. These are the rules and prescriptions for practice that shape the individual's sense of their 'role' as represented by others. The students' self-perception as a social–cultural product emerges in conversations about their role ('what is expected of *me*'). These duties are often implicit and may not be readily apparent. The cultural expectations expressed in dialogue with others position the student and shape, but don't necessarily determine, their agency. The rule or role presented in institutional practices describes functional expectations and tasks. This involves both implicit and explicit acts of forced positioning (van Langenhove & Harré 1995). In everyday discursive practice or workplace conversations the students view their lived world, structured by the rule or roles, from the perspective presented to them by the significant others in the institution. They must reach a level of accepted competence in the eyes of the significant others before they can speak for others ('this is what I think *I/we* can do here').

The autobiographic stories that students or novice practitioners and others tell each other in the practice setting are shared stories of their moral capacities. These story-lines position them in the local moral order as being a particular sort of person (proficient, feeble, sympathetic, antipathetic and so on). In a professional community of practice these stories can be used to identify how they have or will construct knowledge from the available resources or rules. Autobiography is therefore central to personal and professional identity formation, in addition to the maintenance and transformation of communities of practice.

However the model suggests institutional transformation is only possible when an agent is able to speak with the authority of that community. The conversations of the community provide the public psychological spaces in which students or novice practitioners publish or present themselves and are confirmed or rejected (Fig 4.3). It is here that the professionals test what knowledge, both of themselves as well as their world, is valued, how it changes and how new knowledge is created, and how knowledge is used in practice (Higgs et al 2004). Professional education thus becomes a lifelong process of construction of embodied knowledge, which needs to be built on a dialogical model through all stages.

Figure 4.4 illustrates how the agential self can transform professional culture. Cultural maintenance and transformation is brought about through discursive action by human agency. Through conversations and cultural appropriation, the student or novice acting agentially reposition themselves and transform their practice. Difficulties arise when novices are unable to appropriate meanings and are unable to publish their understanding. This is the move from the personal to the public (see Fig 4.3).

Conclusion

The clinician–supervisor is in an important position of observing the professional emergence of a student. To facilitate this process, we claim that they should speak for their community and their profession. The main tool the supervisor needs to use is their conversation. Through conversation with students, supervisors are able to make the culture of the profession explicit for the student and clarify how the rules and practices are historically situated and located within the community. Given these broader roles, supervisors need to become skilled in assisting the students to understand different meanings, to be challenged and to reposition themselves within the learning framework. This requires supervisors to affirm the students' discourse, to encourage them to express alternatives presented by different understandings and perspectives, and to allow them to be comfortable with their individual skills of discourse.

In this chapter, we have argued that the clinical conversation is the basic social reality in which both the student and the profession may relate and develop. We contend that the future capacities of health professions will be greatly influenced by how they initiate new members into their conversations and stories, and engage them in communities of practice.

References

Austin J 1959 How to do things with words. Oxford University Press, UK
Bateson G 1979 Mind and nature. Ballantine, New York
Bhaskar R 1993 Dialectics: The pulse of freedom. Verso, London
Clandinen J, Connelly M 1987 Teachers' personal practical knowledge: what counts as personal in studies of the personal. Journal of Curriculum Studies 19:487–500
Davies B, Harré R 1990 Positioning: the discursive production of selves. Journal for the Theory of Social Behaviour 20:43–63

Dewey J 1933 How we think: a restatement of the relation of reflective thinking to the educative process. DC Heath, Chicago

Ewing R, Smith D 2001 Doing, knowing, being and becoming: the nature of professional practice. In: Higgs J, Titchen A (eds) Professional practice in health, education and the creative arts. Blackwell Science, Oxford, p 16–28

Eraut M 1985 Knowledge creation and knowledge use in professional contexts. Studies in Higher Education 10:117–133

Gustavsson B 2004 Revisiting the philosophical roots of practical knowledge. In: Higgs J, Richardson B, Abrandt-Dahlghren MD (eds) Developing practice knowledge for health professionals. Butterworth-Heinemann, Edinburgh

Harré R, van Langenhove L 1999 Positioning theory. Blackwell, Oxford

Harré R, Moghaddam FM 2003 The self and others. Praeger, Westport CT

Higgs J, Fish D, Rothwell R 2004 Practice knowledge: critical appreciation. In: Higgs J, Richardson B, Abrandt-Dahlghren MD (eds) Developing practice knowledge for health professionals. Butterworth-Heinemann, Edinburgh, p 89–105

Muhlhausler P, Harré R 1990 Pronouns and people: the linguistic construction of social and personal identity. Blackwell, Oxford

Niemi P 1997 Medical students' professional identity: self-reflection during the preclinical years. Medical Education 31:408–415

Phillips D, Fawns R, Hayes B 2002 From personal reflection to social positioning: the development of a transformational model of professional education in midwifery. Nursing Inquiry 9(4):239–249

Pickering M 1990 The supervisory process: an experienced interpersonal relationships and personal growth. National Student Speech Language Hearing Association Journal 17:17–28

Polanyi M 1969 Knowing and being. In: Green M (ed) Learning and being. Routledge & Kegan, London

Ratner C 2000 Agency and culture. Journal for the Theory of Social Behaviour 30:413–433

Reason P, Heron J 1986 Research with people: the paradigm of cooperative experiential enquiry. Person-Centred Review 1:457–476

Richardson B 1999 Professional development: professional knowledge and situated learning in the workplace. Physiotherapy 85:467–473

Schatzki T 2003 The new social ontology. Philosophy of the Social Sciences 33(2):174–202

Schein EH 1978 Career, dynamics: matching individual and organisational needs. Addison-Wesley, Reading MA

Schön D 1983 The reflective practitioner: how professionals think in action. Basic Books, New York

Schön D 1987 Educating the reflective practitioner. Jossey-Bass, London

van Langenhove L, Harré R 1995 Cultural stereotypes and positioning theory. Journal for the Theory of Social Behaviour 24:359–372

Vygotsky LS 1962 Thought and language. trans E Hanfmann & G Vakar. MIT Press, Cambridge MA

Webb G 2004 Clinical education in physiotherapy: a discursive model. PhD in Education thesis. University of Melbourne

Wenger E 1998 Communities of practice: learning, meaning and identity. Cambridge University Press, UK

Williams P 1998 Using theories of professional knowledge and reflective practice to influence educational change. Medical Teacher 20:28–34

Wittgenstein L 1953 Philosophical investigations, 2nd edn. Blackwell, Oxford

Wolcott HF 1988 Ethnographic research in education. In: Jaeger RN (ed) Complementary methods for research in education. Educational Research Association, Washington, p 187–209

CHAPTER 5

Interprofessional education: sharing the wealth

Megan Davidson, Robyn Smith and Nick Stone

THEORIES

The underlying theories in this chapter include the concept of practice epistemology or knowing the nature and source of knowledge that underpins discipline-specific knowledge. Having this deep knowledge provides a foundation to, in turn, develop perspectives and knowledge of other disciplines. A second theoretical construct underpinning this chapter concerns the pedagogy of clinical learning. The authors implicitly rely on a framework of workplace learning, where students are encouraged to acknowledge diversity in approaches to healthcare and to learn in teams including situations that replicate the realities of the clinical setting.

USING THEORIES TO INFORM CURRICULUM DESIGN AND RESEARCH

When designing clinical education curricula using the tenets of interprofessional education (IPE), attention should be paid to the practice epistemologies of a range of healthcare professions. From this basis, differences and similarities can be identified to inform ways of combining and collaborating in IPE. Including IPE as a component of clinical education not only represents a philosophical commitment to embracing diversity of practices within education programs, it also requires detailed planning and timetable coordination in order to ensure it is embedded within the pedagogical framework of health professional education.

USING THEORIES TO DRIVE EDUCATION METHODS

Example: When setting an IPE learning task, the task and learning outcome should be tailored to specific interprofessional practice goals. Low-relevance IPE activities tend to be more passive and decontextualised from applied settings (e.g. combining different professions in a lecture format). High-relevance activities occur when students undertake learning tasks that are more representative of future professional situations.

These include problem-based learning tutorials, using clinical simulation and fostering a team-based collaborative approach to patient assessment and management in the clinical setting. Cross-discipline supervision, such as a nurse educator supervising medical and/or physiotherapy students, is a further example of a teaching method that models interprofessional understanding and practice.

Introduction

This chapter addresses some important questions associated with understanding and implementing interprofessional education (IPE) in clinical and other applied settings. The chapter is divided into three sections to assist readers to review this broad topic. Section 1 covers the history and provides some definitions of IPE, including some rationales for those definitions. In this section, questions are asked such as: Why is IPE needed? What are some defining features of IPE programs? What evidence is there that they 'work'? In Section 2 some examples of research are presented. They focus on ways to judge the effectiveness of interprofessional programs. A typology of IPE outcomes is applied to analyse some of the reported effects of two Australian case studies. In Section 3 some of the perceived and other barriers to implementing IPE are discussed. This also includes some suggested responses to these challenges, and describes enabling factors that have been useful in building successful IPE programs in the clinical or fieldwork context.

Section 1   History and definitions
A very brief history of IPE

Interprofessional practice in the health professions has existed for millennia. The issue of professional fragmentation is also an old, even ancient, issue. Herodotus (c446 BC, 1954 translation) described this of the Egyptians:

> The practice of medicine they split up into separate parts, each doctor being responsible for the treatment of only one disease. There are, in consequence, innumerable doctors ... (p 160)

Abdel-Halim (2006) cites Arabic documents from 1000 years ago that demonstrate the benefits of teamwork in the interests of the patient. More recently, two decades ago the World Health Organization (WHO 1988) formally recognised the need for greater interprofessional education and practice:

> During certain periods of their education students of different health professions learn together the skills necessary for solving the priority health problems of individuals and communities that are known to be particularly amenable to team-work. The emphasis is on learning how to interact with one another. (p 5)

Interestingly, the WHO is currently reviewing global progress towards the goals outlined in its 1988 report (Yan et al 2007). The impetus for the review and the reason for increased attention to IPE are the worldwide shortage and maldistribution of healthcare workers, and the need for better collaboration to maximise the effectiveness of scarce human and other resources.

While some core themes in IPE seem to be timeless, the challenge for current educators and practitioners is to bring IPE in from the margins of their respective curricula. This means a systematic and explicit focus on key elements of IPE in the design, delivery, assessment, research and evaluation associated with health and social care programs.

Of course, for this to happen there must also be substantial policy shifts along with corresponding funding and resourcing arrangements (Stone 2007).

What is IPE?

Agreeing on shared meanings is particularly important when there is a need to collaborate on the design, delivery, assessment and evaluation of programs that involve unfamiliar and possibly 'fuzzy' terms and concepts. A range of divergent terms has been used in the interprofessional area (Table 5.1).

PREFIXES	ADJECTIVES
Multi- Inter- Trans- Cross- Pan-	professional disciplinary

Table 5.1 Range of terms used to describe IPE

In recent research in Victoria, Australia, Stone and Curtis (2007) found that there was vague understanding of what IPE actually means in practice. One-hundred-and-nine comments from 57 respondents were thematically analysed, and the key IPE components of (a) teamwork, collaboration and/or interprofessional practice, and (b) community and/or patient care were identified in only 4.6% and 8.3% of comments respectively.

Use of the term 'interprofessional' is not confined to the domain of health. It is also used to refer to broader sets of vocational areas that are recognised as benefiting from active and systematic interaction and collaboration. School education, theology, law and the justice system, for example, are areas that are clearly important in achieving social and health improvement (Snyder 1987). Nor is it a big leap to include professions relating to the social and health impacts of natural and built environments, such as environmental science, architecture and engineering (Illinois Institute of Technology 2008). It is important to understand the interrelatedness of traditionally separate departments, disciplines and sectors, because their interdependence means that collaboration is often the only way that affordable, lasting, positive change can be effected (Graycar 2008). Our focus here is more modest, and we will limit our scope to the health and social care professions.

While the World Health Organization (1988) originally used the term 'multiprofessional' education (MPE), it has since adopted the more accurate term 'interprofessional' education (IPE) (Yan et al 2007), which has a clear emphasis on interaction between professions, rather than just the 'presence of many'. It is important to distinguish between these terms because MPE now commonly refers to two or more professions learning side-by-side for whatever reason (Barr 2002). Sometimes the terms 'common learning' and 'shared learning' are also used to describe situations in which students from different disciplines are co-located, but may not necessarily purposefully interact.

A widely agreed international definition of IPE is: 'Occasions when two or more professions learn *with, from and about* each other to improve collaboration and the quality of care' (Freeth et al 2005, p xv).

The 'with, from and about' are important aspects that are often omitted from educational activities labelled 'IPE' but which, in fact, more closely resemble 'MPE'. IPE can also be seen as a subset of the broader construct 'interprofessional learning' (IPL), which includes any sort of interprofessional experience where learning may occur, such as informal and unplanned activities at any stage before, during or after initial qualification. Barr et al (2005) offer the following definition: 'IPL is learning arising from interaction between members (or students) of two or more professions either as a product of interprofessional education or happening spontaneously' (p xxiii).

Why IPE and IPP?

There are many pressing imperatives for more and better IPE, based on assumptions involving two causal steps:
1 IPE will lead to better interprofessional practice (IPP) and, in turn, that
2 IPP will lead to better health outcomes for clients, patients and communities.

There are also convincing arguments and some research to suggest that improvements in IPP are associated with higher levels of job morale and satisfaction among health professionals (Barr et al 2005, Day et al 2006, DeLoach 2003, Reeves et al 2008). One could logically assume that improved work morale and satisfaction should lead to better recruitment and retention. It should not be surprising that improving IPP offers a range of benefits in addition to improved patient or client care. It has been known for some time that establishing successful teamwork features, such as respectful and fair relationships, and explicitly understood roles and responsibilities, is likely to increase productivity, a sense of control, personal health and well being, and a lower risk of 'unhealthy' occupational stress among staff (see, for example, Ferrie 2004, Hackman & Oldham 1976, Karasek, 1979).

There is considerable evidence that IPE can, at least in the short term, positively affect a range of traits associated with effective IPP, such as related knowledge, skills and attitudes (Zwarenstein et al 2005). There is also a growing evidence base that effective IPP can improve health outcomes for a range of health conditions, most notably those that are chronic and complex. So while we can be confident that IPE achieves acquisition of relevant knowledge, skills and attitudes, and possibly this in turn improves IPP, the causal link between IPE and improved patient outcomes has not yet been fully demonstrated (Fig 5.1). Given the complexity of the system in which professional education occurs this link may prove extremely difficult to demonstrate, and research effort may be better expended on further exploring the role of interprofessional *practice* rather than IPE in improving patient outcomes.

Given the number of complex, interacting, social systems involved in IPE and IPP, it will take an extraordinary commitment of research resources, probably sustained for over a decade or more, to establish the burden of proof typically expected when working within hypothetico-deductive methodological frameworks. Such research might involve, for example, tracking large cohorts of students who (a) do and (b) do not engage in IPE during their professional preparation. They would need to be assessed at a number of stages to monitor their interprofessional development and, eventually, to evaluate the impact of this learning, first on their professional practice, and second on patient and/or community health measures. Even if such support was available for this sort of research, it would be extremely challenging to disentangle potentially confounding effects at various points in the related nomological network. Therefore, it seems unlikely that traditional bio-medical research models will be practicable in evaluating the effects of IPE and IPP, and that more eclectic, interdisciplinary and mixed-method approaches may be needed (Stone 2006b).

For the positive influence between IPE, IPP and health outcomes to be established (in Australia at least), there first needs to be significant change such that there are supportive policies and recurrent funding to instigate and support the integration and maintenance of IPE into health courses. Once this prerequisite is addressed, ensuing reform and other positive changes will require sustained support for the necessary research and evaluation

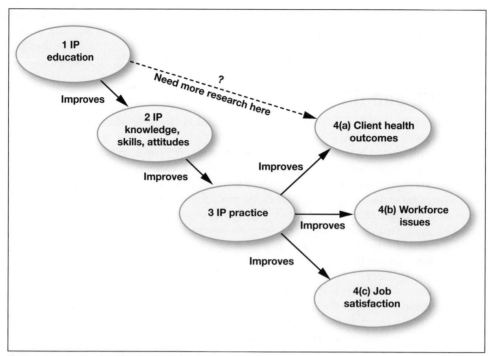

Figure 5.1 The proposed outcomes of IPE

to establish a substantial IPE and IPP evidence base. International experience suggests that this requires multilateral partnerships between stakeholders, such as universities, governments, service providers, and relevant consumer and professional bodies.

Box 5.1 summarises some of the main drivers for better interprofessional approaches to healthcare.

BOX 5.1 Forces for mainstreaming interprofessional approaches

- An ageing population with complex health and support needs and associated costs
- Chronic diseases (including 'lifestyle' diseases) demanding a greater proportion of healthcare resources
- Workforce redesign (e.g. devolution of some healthcare responsibilities traditionally the domain of GPs to other health professionals)
- Healthcare moving from acute to community-based or ambulatory and domiciliary settings
- The shortage of medical, nursing and other health professionals, especially in rural and outer-urban areas
- Expectation that patients and carers will be active partners in their healthcare
- Increased recognition of the importance of preventative approaches, health promotion and education to optimise self-management potential
- Recognition of benefits of IPP for patient health outcomes and health professionals' job satisfaction

- Increased accountability and demands by patients–public for greater transparency, quality and safety in healthcare
- Need to maximise efficiency in public and private spending, and reduce duplication of health communication, treatments and procedures
- The necessity in rural and remote areas for non-medical professionals to perform a wider range of 'medical' procedures
- Societal trends towards greater democratisation and egalitarianism in workplaces
- Recognition of the need for greater continuity of care versus episodic intervention
- A need to address fragmentation of various health system levels, responsibilities and processes
- Need to improve cost effectiveness of education and professional development by identifying common learning and training needs, sharing resources and teaching expertise.

What does IPE look like?

IPE occurs when two or more professions learn 'with, from and about each other'. The context for this learning is the fostering of collaborative practice and improved quality of care. Learning activities can be evaluated in terms of relevance and suitability to IPE (Table 5.2). Low-relevance activities, such as lectures, tend to be more passive and decontextualised from applied settings, while high-relevance activities occur where students undertake learning tasks that are closer to professional life.

ACTIVITY	EVALUATION OF RELEVANCE TO IPE
Lectures	Limited scope for interprofessional interaction and its assessment; may be appropriate for delivery of knowledge-based components and content about other professional roles, the need for and principles of interprofessional practice, teamwork, collaboration, supporting research, models, issues, international developments. Traditionally passive, but interactive–experiential large-group teaching methods are emerging that better support IPE.
Practical/applied or lab-based learning	High experiential value (usually has a technical skills-acquisition focus) but may have limited opportunities for interaction between students. Can be structured to incorporate different disciplines working together to acquire or practise a specific skill.
Tutorial	Can range from low to high experiential components. Scope for student interaction, and its assessment varies in proportion to how active or passive the teaching strategies are: pure listening, reading and writing vs discussion, self-directed, inquiry, problem or case-based learning, simulation or role-play. Tutorial-based learning can be highly effective as a way of exploring interprofessional approaches.
Online learning	May involve individual learning and group activities with varying levels of interaction depending on design of the unit. Interaction is limited to a 'virtual' environment and may be experienced by students as too divorced from the 'real world' to provide a highly effective interprofessional learning experience.

➡

➡

ACTIVITY	EVALUATION OF RELEVANCE TO IPE
Simulation	Some simulation environments (e.g. emergency care) are 'high fidelity' in their ability to simulate actual clinical environments and provide realistic opportunities for team-based patient care. Simulation can be structured to incorporate different disciplines working together to acquire or practise a specific skill (e.g. physiotherapy, medical and nursing students learning together in a simulated setting to manage aspects of cardiorespiratory patient care).
e-clinics	Opportunities to observe recorded or real-time patient—professional interactions and team interactions. When combined with collaborative, experiential small-group or tutorial opportunities provides learning opportunities for IPE.
Fieldwork	Ranges from work shadowing (observational) to practice under supervision. Opportunities for IPL may be structured or incidental. There is significant potential for structured IPE opportunities where students share patients, complete joint assessments, engage in collaborative group problem solving and interactive discussion of the process of teamwork and IP clinical care.

Table 5.2 Range of learning activities evaluated with relevance to IPE

The matrix shown in Table 5.3 has proven useful in planning programs and learning activities as students progress through their courses, for example, by incrementally increasing relevance of experiences as they develop more professional levels of associated competence. It also offers a clarification of terms, especially the difference between 'multi' and interprofessional education.

	MONO-DISCIPLINARY	CROSS-DISCIPLINARY TEACHING–CONTENT	MULTI-PROFESSIONAL	INTER-PROFESSIONAL (IDEALLY)
Shared learning spaces or activities	no	no	yes	yes
Some content from other disciplines	no	possible	possible	yes
Some teachers from other disciplines	no	possible	possible	yes
Learning about roles of other professions	no	possible	possible	yes
Focus on collabora-tion– teamwork	possible	possible	possible	yes
Focus on improving healthcare	possible	possible	possible	yes
Students from different disciplines deliberately interact	no	no	possible	yes
IP student interaction– teamwork is formally assessed	no	no	no	yes

Table 5.3 Matrix of program features with various degrees of 'interprofessionality'

In the shorter term, it seems unlikely that all of the 'ideal' IPE conditions in the right-hand column (Table 5.3) can be addressed at once in most settings. However, using this schema as a guide may assist with forward planning based on the principle that the more of these features that can be provided, the greater the likelihood of durable and transferable learning taking place.

As can be seen from the examples in Tables 5.2 and 5.3, there are many possible IPE pathways that can evolve from the complex systems typically involved in preparation for practice and continuing professional development within the health workforce. Rather than replacing or imposing further layers upon existing programs, IPE requires adjusting *how* these programs unfold, while still addressing important extant discipline-specific learning outcomes. While some elements of existing 'model' programs may be borrowed, or more likely adapted, it would be very difficult to transplant a program intact from one setting to another. Some have been inspired by exemplary practice, such as the Southampton New Generation Project (O'Halloran et al 2006), and sought to use it as a blueprint. However, the learning and practice context and the relationships are important success factors in IPE. Therefore direct application of an existing program risks early failure if it is not adapted to fit well with local practice and does not involve the local stakeholders in the development process. The ACT Interprofessional Learning Project is an example of a health department-led initiative (Box 5.2) and the Southampton New Generation Project (Box 5.3) is an example of a university-led IPE program. It should be noted that both projects required substantial financial and human resources in their development and implementation phases.

BOX 5.2 The ACT Interprofessional Learning Project

The Australian Capital Territory encompasses the environs of the national capital, Canberra. The ACT IPL project aims to establish and grow an interprofessional culture in healthcare in the ACT. The project commenced with a comprehensive review of the literature (Braithwaite & Travaglia 2005) and a series of discussion papers and, subsequently, an IPL framework and implementation plan. The plan encompasses the health authority (ACT Health), healthcare facilities, education institutions, professional bodies, healthcare teams, managers and professionals. IPL at a pre- and post-qualification stage, at an individual and organisational level, is the target of the project.

This project is an example of a system-wide approach to IPE and IPP. It shows how leadership and resources from the local health authority with strong involvement of education stakeholders has achieved a commitment to achieving a shift in the culture of healthcare and health education toward interprofessional approaches.

Online. Available: http://health.act.gov.au/c/health?a=sp&did=10153142 accessed 18 Dec 2008

In terms of how a particular discipline relates to another there are also a range of possibilities and models, such as:

- a common foundation year (usually mandatory)
- shared fieldwork and/or clinical education placements
- shared classes
- shared experiential activities
- community-development oriented activities.

BOX 5.3 The Southampton New Generation Project

In 2005 the Universities of Southampton and Portsmouth embarked on a project that now incorporates a number of short IPE experiences into the curricula of fourteen disciplines. Students undertake three units of interprofessional learning across their program (O'Halloran et al 2006). The first unit introduces students to team roles and teamwork. The second unit involves a clinical audit task and further development of collaborative teamwork skills. In the third unit student teams undertake a service improvement project requiring them to engage in interprofessional problem solving. Unit 1 is based at the university campus while Units 2 and 3 are fieldwork based.

Online. Available: http://www.commonlearning.net/ Accessed 18 Dec 2008

Through most of these offerings there is a variable degree to which students share their curriculum. At one extreme they might work together on assignments or projects, but only focus and be assessed on aspects uniquely associated with their own discipline. At the other extreme they may share common objectives, roles and assessment requirements. In the middle, of course, there may be scope for both shared and discipline-specific components. This is often seen as the most appropriate approach as it identifies common content, values and approaches while recognising that all health team members do not have identical skill sets, roles and responsibilities.

'Clinical education' and the interprofessional context

Historically the term 'clinical education' has mostly been used to refer to supervised experience in any setting providing direct healthcare services, such as hospitals and clinics. Many professions, however, work in other settings, such as education, welfare and community service settings. Indeed healthcare is increasingly delivered in sub-acute and community settings rather than acute hospitals, although much health professional education has yet to adjust to this reality (Nair & Finucane 2003). 'Professional experience', 'professional placement' and 'fieldwork' are terms used to describe student placements more broadly in the range of clinical and non-clinical settings. In the remainder of this chapter we focus predominantly on discussion of interprofessional approaches to education–learning that occur in the applied context of service delivery—that is on fieldwork or clinical education activities.

In section 2, we describe two examples of fieldwork-based IPE from the Australian context.

Section 2   Examples of interprofessional clinical education
A typology for interprofessional education outcomes

One of the challenges in reviewing examples of interprofessional clinical education is the range of evaluation approaches and outcome measures used in the field. Barr et al (2005, p 43) extended the 1967 Kirkpatrick four-level classification of educational outcomes (Reaction, Learning, Behaviour, Results) to a six-level typology of outcomes for application to IPE:

- Level 1: Reaction
- Level 2a: Modification of attitudes–perceptions
- Level 2b: Acquisition of knowledge and skills
- Level 3: Behavioural change
- Level 4a: Change in organisational practice
- Level 4b: Benefits to patients–clients.

The suggested typology allows program evaluators and researchers to explicitly select the particular outcomes of interest, and to report those outcomes in a way that will allow meaningful comparisons between programs and studies. The benefits to learners are largely confined to levels 1, 2a, 2b and 3.

Level 1 Reactions are the learner's responses to the experience. This could include the extent to which students found the IPE experience enjoyable, engaging, satisfying or meaningful. Evaluation of Level 1 outcomes generally occurs at the end of the IPE experience. Level 2a Modification of attitudes and perceptions involves the measurement before and after the IPE of attitudes towards other health professions and towards interprofessional collaboration and teamwork. Level 2b Acquisition of knowledge and skills would be demonstrated by evaluating the learners' understanding of the roles and responsibilities of other professions, their knowledge of interprofessional practice and the nature of teamwork. Level 3 Behavioural change is the observed transfer of learning to a practice setting, and may involve observed or self-reported changes in interprofessional communication and collaboration behaviours and in improved links between professions and teams.

Level 4a Change in organisational practice involves impacts at the level of the organisation and the systems of care delivery. Examples are structural changes to the way healthcare teams are organised or managed, and changes to the level, type or mix of services available to patients. Level 4b Benefits to patients or clients include improvements in aspects of health and wellbeing, or their satisfaction with care.

In their review of 107 IPE studies, Barr et al (2005, p 75) found that the most commonly reported outcomes were Level 1, 4a and 2b and that few studies reported Level 3 or 4b outcomes. The review included pre and post-registration IPE conducted at universities, in practice settings and at both.

Davidson et al (2008) systematically reviewed studies reporting interprofessional education in a clinical or fieldwork setting. The review included 25 reports of pre-registration interprofessional education in a fieldwork setting. The IPE experience ranged from 2.5 hours to 9 weeks, with the most common being of 2 weeks' duration. Team size ranged from two to ten with up to 14 disciplines included (median 3). Medicine and nursing were most commonly included as part of the IP team; physiotherapy and occupational therapy were the most frequently included allied health disciplines.

Outcomes of the fieldwork IPE experiences were typically evaluated by questionnaires and focus groups. Limitations of the studies were that about half gave little detail as to how outcomes data were analysed, and few used rigorous strategies such as data triangulation or controlled for interviewer or social desirability biases. Failure to use standardised assessment instruments with evidence for reliability and validity is a feature of the field, with researchers tending to invent one-off scales to measure change in attitude, knowledge, and skills before and after the IPE. Qualitative evaluations, for example by focus groups and interviews, are widely used in studies but frequently are not conducted by an independent assessor. These study limitations are likely to result in an overestimate of the benefits of the IPE experiences. Keeping in mind these limitations of the evidence, let us take a closer look at the benefits to learners of clinical–fieldwork IPE by examining two Australian projects.

Case 1: The Rural Interprofessional Education (RIPE) project

The RIPE project was funded by the Department of Human Services in Victoria and involved all universities in that state. There were two major objectives: to develop and implement an undergraduate interprofessional learning program; and to provide the opportunity for students to have a positive experience of rural health work and life. The latter objective was clearly aimed at raising interest in returning to rural healthcare, either during further training or post-registration. The project was evaluated primarily via pre- and post-placement questionnaires that included short, written responses and a range of rating scale items. These data were augmented with other qualitative sources such as reflective records, online discussion and tutorial transcripts, observation and discussion during tutorials, and informal feedback from students, preceptors and coordinators. Throughout these processes, there was a concerted focus on self-assessment and structured reflection as a means of developing the self-awareness capabilities important to effective IP practice.

Over five years, a total of 140 students, primarily from medicine and nursing with a small number of physiotherapy and pharmacy students, undertook two-week placements in rural health services across regional and rural Victoria, the most south eastern state in mainland Australia. Students from a wide range of backgrounds—including about 25% international students—volunteered through an expression of interest form to go on placement in one of four geographic regions across the state. Most medical students participated in their own time, and few received formal credit towards their course requirements. Most nursing, pharmacy and physiotherapy students did receive formal credit, usually as a component of their total rural and/or clinical placement requirements. They were allocated to groups of two to four students from different disciplines, depending on site capacity. They took part in a pre-departure briefing, mostly by teleconference, to clarify expectations and logistics such as transport and accommodation, and to initiate rapport building within the group.

On the first day of the placement, they met at the most convenient site in their geographical region for the first tutorial. This consisted of structured activities designed to: introduce some key aspects of interprofessional practice and teamwork, familiarise them with the placement components, discuss expectations of key stakeholders, anticipate and plan for possible problems, and further develop effective working relationships. The main components of the program were:

- clinical and community-based activities and projects
- participating regularly in an online discussion forum
- a mid-placement review involving all students and preceptors and
- preparing to present their projects at the final tutorial.

During the placement students shared designated preceptors for each discipline and, wherever possible, worked together throughout the fortnight. They undertook community and practice-based learning that ranged from observation (work shadowing) to more hands-on activities such as patient history taking and assessment, minor procedures and home visits. There was a strong emphasis on interaction with the local community, both informally through social and recreational activities, as well as more organised events such as presentations to local service and other community organisations. The major collaborative task was to identify and complete a small community-based project. This usually involved community consultation and needs analysis. Each project was designed to boost local community capacity to manage its own health, and was presented at the second tutorial at the end of the placement. This tutorial also included a structured debriefing, reflective discussion, and identification of strategies and opportunities to continue IPL into the future.

Detailed outcomes have at this stage only been published for the first three years ($n = 91$) of the project (McNair et al 2005). A sample of findings below includes the final aggregate results ($n = 140$) from two years later. They are reported using the evaluation typology developed by Barr et al (2005). A more detailed account of this research is forthcoming.

LEVEL 1:   REACTION
High levels of satisfaction with the placement (sustained at 12 months) were identified among the participation students. Positive evaluation of preceptors and positive ratings of IP learning were achieved.

LEVEL 2A: MODIFICATION OF ATTITUDES–PERCEPTIONS
Pre-placement medical students were less likely than nursing or allied health (AH) students to anticipate being active team members. Nursing and AH students were more confident in their own interprofessional effectiveness. Pre- to post-placement change: students had more positive attitudes toward nurses undertaking traditionally GP roles ($p = 0.008$); increased agreement that IPE should be a core part of undergraduate training ($p = 0.001$); and feeling respected by the other profession improved ($p < 0.001$). Pre- and post-test levels of respect for other disciplines were high.

LEVEL 2B: ACQUISITION OF KNOWLEDGE AND SKILLS
The study identified significant positive change ($p < 0.001$) in knowledge and under-standing of roles. Self-rating of own interprofessional skills decreased post-test ($p < 0.001$, from 'strongly agree' to 'agree'). Females were more likely to agree they would and had developed interprofessional skills during placement (pre-test $p = 0.028$, post-test $p = 0.003$). There was a high pre- and post-test agreement about the importance of interprofessional practice; and an increase in beliefs about the positive impact of interprofessional approaches on patient health outcomes ($p = 0.040$).

LEVEL 3:   BEHAVIOURAL CHANGE
There was significant pre-post improvement on the item 'I felt like I was an active member of a multiprofessional team' ($p < 0.001$). Significant improvement was also observed pre-post in self-confidence in interprofessional collaboration ($p < 0.001$) and in interacting with students and practitioners (both $p < 0.001$) of other professions.

The RIPE project focused on Levels 1–3 of the typology and identified major shifts at the levels of learner reaction, modification of attitudes and perceptions, acquisition of knowledge and skills, and some evidence of behavioural change—from self-assessed questionnaire completion. The results indicate that students significantly improved essential skills, knowledge and attitudes that are associated with effective IPP. Along with findings from follow-up data (collected an average of 12 months later), the program appears to have had lasting positive effects on these students IPE.

Case 2:   La Trobe University–Northern Health Allied Health project
The 'Learning Together to Work Together' project was funded by the Department of Human Services in Victoria. This collaborative project between a university and a metropolitan health service focused on the clinical education experience of students on placement in the health service.

Twenty-two final year Allied Health students from five disciplines, occupational therapy, physiotherapy, podiatry, social work and speech pathology, were placed in a number of acute and subacute settings in teams of three or four with the IPE experience scheduled over a four-week period. Activities included facilitated small group discussion, case-related meetings, and collaborative patient assessment and management. Clinical placements were offered in adult general medicine, inpatient aged-care assessment and management, falls and balance out-patient program, paediatric out-patients, women's and children's inpatient services and the Emergency Department. Outcome evaluation was by way of focus groups and interviews with students, facilitators, clinical educators and patients after the placement, and by administration before and after the program of the Interdisciplinary Education Perception Scale (IEPS) (Luecht et al 1990). Focus groups and interviews were conducted by a project coordinator or one of the project management team not directly involved in teaching the students. Transcripts of the focus groups and interviews were analysed by two independent assessors using the Barr et al (2005) typology of outcomes (Smith et al 2007).

LEVEL 1: REACTION
Based on student reports, the IPE experience across most clinical areas provided an excellent opportunity for students to work collaboratively with patients and as a team to see a patient through their episode of care. The students reported positive benefit from the direct experience of each other's roles and from the opportunity to witness a patient achieving tangible health benefits and outcomes. The students commonly attributed the observed patient outcomes to collaborative team intervention. The students who participated in the Care Coordination–Emergency Department placement had fewer opportunities to share patients, and the perceived benefit was lower for this group. Students enjoyed the opportunity to meet other students from different disciplines and various placements. Although some of the students did not share patients directly, they were able to contribute in discussion time and draw on differing experiences. The students reported positive benefit from learning from one another when brought together for facilitated small group discussion, in addition to opportunities to reflect on their own interprofessional practice when in the balance of the placement.

LEVEL 2A: MODIFICATION OF ATTITUDES–PERCEPTIONS
The IEPS provided some insights into interprofessional perceptions. The IEPS comprises eighteen statements about one's own and other health professions answered on a six-level agreement scale from 'strongly agree' to 'strongly disagree'. In this study the IEPS total score was calculated as the sum of the item scores, and a higher score indicated less positive attitudes. Students' perceptions of their own and other professions were positive at the beginning of the IEPS (mean 23.91, sd 5.69) and changed in a positive direction at the end of the IEPS experience (mean 20.14, sd 6.58). The difference was significant (t-test, $p = 0.048$) and the change of 3.77 points appears to be an important difference. Item 6 'Individuals in my profession need to cooperate with other professions' had the most positive pre-test mean (0.55). The largest positive change occurred in item 4 'Individuals in other professions respect the work done by my profession'.

LEVEL 2B: ACQUISITION OF KNOWLEDGE AND SKILLS
In terms of knowledge and skills, a strong theme that emerged was students' improved understanding of other disciplines and their roles. This was described as greater depth of knowledge, greater appreciation of others' skills and contribution, and improved knowledge about why, when and how to refer to or draw on other health professionals.

LEVEL 3:   BEHAVIOURAL CHANGE

There was evidence of student behaviour change during the placement. IPE facilitators, discipline supervisors and university clinical coordinators all observed or reported changes in student behaviour that reflected improved capacity for interprofessional practice. Follow-up phone calls to students post-graduation indicated that the majority of students had used their project participation as part of their job application process. All students contacted felt that participation in the project had increased their work readiness, citing examples of improved confidence working in teams, deeper understanding of how teams function, and strengthened communication and interaction with others. Of those who were working at the time of the follow-up phone calls (six students), four quoted direct examples of applying their IPCE knowledge as new graduates and a further two perceived that their project experience would be beneficial in future work.

LEVEL 4A: CHANGE IN ORGANISATIONAL PRACTICE

Organisational change was noted with the introduction of funding for a small amount of podiatry time based on the experience of the IPE project. Reorienting the health service clinical placement program to foster ongoing interprofessional collaboration and learning opportunities was another clear organisational outcome of the project.

LEVEL 4B: BENEFITS TO PATIENTS–CLIENTS

Patients interviewed for the study reported positive experiences of the IPE program. No formal comparison was made of patient outcomes compared with those treated by students not participating in the program.

The developmental 'Learning Together to Work Together' project endeavoured to consider results across the full spectrum of the outcomes framework. It provided pre-post and qualitative information for the groups who participated in the program but did not formally assess patient outcomes. This was an iterative project with the final interprofessional clinical education model comprising one 3.5-hour facilitated learning session followed by seven 2-hour sessions with follow-up tasks, shared patients and clinical experience. Further research is needed to compare different models and intensities of interprofessional clinical education activity in order to better understand which approaches are most effective in achieving learning objectives across the whole outcomes framework.

In Section 1 we indicated that the impetus driving the growing interest in IPE and IPP by government, healthcare and education is based largely on trends in population demographics, burden of chronic illness and workforce considerations. Although the endpoint of greatest interest is the safety, quality and efficiency of patient care, there also appears to be personal benefits to healthcare professionals who work in supportive interprofessional teams. In this section, we have outlined the positive benefits to students of IPE experiences and provided two examples of interprofessional clinical or fieldwork education. In the final section, we will outline the challenges inherent in planning and delivering effective interprofessional clinical or fieldwork education.

Section 3   The barriers and enablers for clinical education across the professions

The World Health Organization (WHO1988) flagged the importance of training health personnel in teams twenty years ago. There appears to be strong validity in the idea of training health professionals in interprofessional practice and, as outlined earlier in this chapter, growing evidence of the benefits to patients, professionals and health systems for doing so. Despite this, single-discipline education continues as the norm in Australia. So what then are the barriers to interprofessional clinical education, and what are the essential elements needed to maximise the likelihood of a sustained and successful fieldwork–clinical IPE program?

There is no universal blueprint for how to 'do' interprofessional clinical education. From the available evidence we can draw common principles and the key components for successful programs, however there is no recipe for an ideal model (Davidson et al 2008). Given that interprofessional clinical education remains novel, fostering this method of learning is a significant exercise in change management. Many of the barriers to and enablers of interprofessional clinical education are those identified in any change management process. Introducing interprofessional clinical education is essentially a process of getting the stakeholders interested in the idea, helping them to shift their practice, then supporting consolidation of the new practice so that this becomes the new norm.

Barriers to interprofessional clinical education

The World Health Organization listed some of the challenges of implementing multiprofessional education (1988, pp 50–1). Twenty years on and many of these issues continue to constrain the implementation of interprofessional learning. A number of the more significant ones are highlighted in this section.

Professional identity and socialisation

There is a body of literature on the development of professional identity, and a great deal of investment by various professions in socialising new inductees into their chosen profession. One of the major challenges to achieving interprofessional education and practice is the belief of some that learning or practising interprofessionally will diminish each discipline's unique professional skill set or identity. Instead of perceiving interprofessional approaches as a potential threat, the capacity to practise interprofessionally needs reframing as a core competency of each health profession. One way to overcome this barrier is by education that promotes the idea that true interprofessional working requires the capacity to understand and value the unique contribution to client care by each professional and to work collaboratively to maximise benefit for the client (Barr et al 2005).

Policy and current practice

Observing current policy and practice provides one way to measure the level of interest in interprofessional learning and practice. Although there has been a significant evolution internationally in interprofessional learning and practice in the past decade in Australia (Department of Health 2001, Curran 2004), the policy framework has really only begun to emerge in the past five years. For example, work commenced on interprofessional learning through ACT Health in 2004, and a recent policy document released in Victoria by the Department of Human Services emphasises the importance of person-centred, interprofessional approaches with older people using healthcare (ACT Health 2008, DHS 2007).

Despite the lack of explicit policy frameworks, some specific practice areas have developed IPP examples that seem to be driven by necessity or the needs of the client group more than by philosophy or policy. For example, rural health, paediatrics, aged care, mental health, community health and palliative care, all have a stronger history of interprofessional approaches. In areas such as rural health, interprofessional practice partly answers the need for peer support and collegial relationships when many professionals are sole practitioners for their discipline, and facilities and staff numbers are smaller, thereby fostering a more collaborative approach. In some areas—aged care, paediatrics and mental health, for example—the needs of the client are complex, and effective care demands greater coordination and collaboration from the treating team. Where these strong drivers for interprofessional collaboration are absent, there is less impetus for change. Still lacking from the Australian system is a cohesive policy agenda to underpin and provide a framework for the many pockets of isolated interprofessional learning and practice occurring across the country.

Structures and logistics

Our system is currently oriented to single discipline models of training, management and practice. While some change is occurring, the majority of training institutions still provide learning in discipline-specific programs with very limited collaborative learning or opportunities for interprofessional education in the university. This plays out in the organisation of clinical education and fieldwork placements. Timing, duration, frequency and focus of fieldwork are often incompatible across the disciplines, rendering almost impossible the task of getting students from different disciplines together in a clinical setting for a meaningful learning experience. This is one of the strongest barriers emerging from the international literature on interprofessional clinical education (Davidson et al 2008). Related to this, registration, supervisory and accountability requirements are usually discipline specific. While this is important to ensure appropriate credentialing and competency to practice, the lack of focus on interprofessionalism as a core competency for each discipline results in limited value being placed on attaining and developing this sophisticated skill set.

The structure of the educational process also influences opportunities for interprofessional clinical education. For example, medical clinical education commonly occurs through the clinical school model where one hospital or health service coordinates and provides the majority of the learning experiences for a cohort of medical students. In contrast, allied health students may have a mix of clinical or fieldwork placements across a number of organisations and in a range of settings. Social work and speech pathology students, for example, may have placements completely outside the health system and the medical model of care. Typically they experience policy settings, community and advocacy organisations and the education system. While this provides many opportunities to these students for interprofessional interaction with other sets of professionals, there are logistics impacts for organising interprofessional learning in healthcare.

Labels

As discussed earlier in this chapter, shared understandings are essential for interprofessional approaches. Although there are widely agreed definitions in the published literature about the differences between multi- and interprofessional learning and practice, the terms are inconsistently used in everyday practice. The terms multi- and interdisciplinary continue to be used interchangeably and incorrectly. Many clinicians believe that they are interprofessional in their approach, when on closer examination practice is multidisciplinary–multiprofessional, missing the essential components of collaborative decision making, interactive teamwork and person centred-ness. Lack of understanding about the notion of learning with, from and about each other for the benefit of the patient or client is a significant barrier to the progress of implementing interprofessional clinical education.

SKILLS VALUED AND MEASURED DIFFERENTLY

Task-related, discipline specific, skill-based competencies are perceived by students, clinicians and academics as vital acquisitions from the fieldwork placement experience. The skills related to working effectively in a team, understanding the process of care, and demonstrating interprofessional competencies are generally perceived as secondary skills. Some would suggest these can be developed post-basic training and are not necessary core competencies for the entry-level practitioner. These perceptions present a significant barrier to fostering interprofessional learning in the fieldwork setting, particularly for entry-level students. If the skill sets for interprofessional working are considered less relevant or important to achieving competence as an entry-level practitioner, there is less impetus to focus on acquiring these skills during the clinical education experience.

Role models and advocates

The limited availability of interprofessional role models and practice exemplars of interprofessional working remains a challenge. Academic and professional staff should model the effective collaborative practice that is the target of interprofessional clinical education. This can be difficult if there are insufficient resources or limited commitment to the changes involved in implementing an interprofessional program. People who are excessively stressed and overworked are unlikely to be effective partners in even the most positive change initiatives. Educators seem sometimes to struggle with the challenges involved in moving towards a stronger interprofessional focus. Complex team interactions and managing care using a person-centred approach requires a greater tolerance of uncertainty and ambiguity compared with more familiar, monodisciplinary practice and learning.

In mainstream healthcare organisations—settings that provide significant numbers of clinical placements to healthcare students—interprofessional practice exists in only limited areas and services. As a result, there are few opportunities for students to directly observe and participate in effective interprofessional teams. Much of the current opportunity for interprofessional learning in the fieldwork setting may come from applying a 'compare and contrast' model rather than providing students with direct experience of effective interprofessional working. Student learning can result from comparing the theory of how interprofessional practice *could* work with what they actually observe in the clinical setting. While this fosters some learning, having positive practice examples and strong interprofessional role models is preferable.

Resourcing

Resourcing is one of the less direct barriers to interprofessional learning. The need for additional resources for interprofessional clinical education is largely a result of the logistic and structural barriers described earlier. While interprofessional learning is being developed, the investment of resources to support change is paramount. However, once established with the organisational and operational hurdles overcome, the demands on teaching and supervision time for interprofessional clinical education are not necessarily higher than would be the case for monodisciplinary placements. Availability of adequate group learning spaces may be an issue in some fieldwork locations.

Enablers to effective interprofessional practice
Foster a positive, collaborative approach to change

Implementing interprofessional clinical education is a change management process, and resistance to change is normal and to be expected. Change requires people to shift from their comfort zone and move from their current practice. Being aware of the elements of the change process and the tools and skills necessary to manage a complex change process will enable more effective implementation of interprofessional clinical education. Given the nature of the structural barriers and the importance of collaboration in interprofessional clinical education, establishing a sense of urgency and a guiding coalition (Kotter 1996) are particularly critical steps for fostering change in this area. Multi-sectoral buy-in from government, universities, hospitals and other agencies, community providers, professional associations, students, consumer advocates and employers is important if interprofessional approaches are to become the norm for fieldwork education.

As for any significant change in practice, institutional support and effective leadership are critical. This may be effectively achieved by establishing a dedicated centre or unit that formally brings together the key stakeholders in a partnership approach to interprofessional clinical education. This may include a number of universities working with one healthcare group, or a number of healthcare and fieldwork agencies working closely with a university that trains different healthcare professionals. Whatever the components of the model, a key factor promoting success is the formal framework for collaboration that enables effective combining of resources, expertise, and professions and shared responsibility for the development, implementation and evaluation of the interprofessional clinical education experience.

Shared language, vision and understanding

When working across disciplines it becomes clear that individual professional stereotypes, myths and misunderstandings can present significant barriers to interprofessional working. Myths and misconceptions need to be addressed systematically and proactively. It is important to work to understand where the anxieties, concerns and resistance are coming from and actively address them. Shared language about interprofessional learning and practice is essential to developing shared understanding and effective working relationships. This in turn fosters development of a shared vision and enables longer-term commitment and planning for interprofessional clinical education.

Provide an authentic, applied fieldwork experience

Students engaging in interprofessional clinical education benefit from learning with, from and about each other. It has been established (from research highlighted in this chapter) that this requires direct experience and observation of each others' work, attitudes, decision-making approaches, clinical reasoning and interventions. However, sharing of the clinical experience can remain a superficial observation unless there are structured opportunities for reflection, discussion and 'unpacking' the *process* of care delivery. Students need to understand and apply in practice the theoretical concepts about how teams work. They need an opportunity to consider how decisions are made; different team roles; how to influence team decisions; how to work as an effective interprofessional team member; and their role and others' roles in fostering person-centred, interprofessional care. While there are many options for delivering these experiences, tailored fieldwork that focuses on technical and clinical skill development as well as on understanding the process of interprofessional care provide an opportunity for a rich experience that better reflects real life. Pragmatics may require that fieldwork be supplemented with online experiences, theoretical exercises or project work. However, students do not necessarily consider these models an effective substitute for robust interprofessional fieldwork experiences (Smith et al 2007).

The amount of interprofessional clinical education needed to deliver a sustained effect is unknown. The literature provides no specific recommendations regarding the timing, frequency, content or intensity of interprofessional clinical education (Davidson et al

2008). The wide range of interprofessional clinical education experiences described in the literature cover everything from a once-off session (Greene et al 1996) to an intensive program in which an interprofessional healthcare student team is responsible for staffing a hospital ward for a period of weeks (Reeves & Freeth 2002). There are examples of transformative experiences occurring even in relatively short periods of time (Stone 2006a). Learning theory, however, suggests that reinforcement and the opportunity to integrate and apply learning on an iterative basis produces effective learning outcomes. Therefore models that provide exposure to interprofessional clinical education over a number of placement settings and over a period of time are more likely to produce sustained outcomes.

Reframe interprofessionalism as a core competency for all disciplines

As with any attempt to develop higher order, general abilities, there is a need to acknowledge this is a long-term endeavour that may take several years to (a) effect significant changes, and (b) fully discern the positive outcomes that result. The likelihood of students transferring their interprofessional learning into workplaces increases with multiple and logically sequenced opportunities to collaborate with other health professionals and students on meaningful tasks. For these opportunities to occur, interprofessional skills need to be described and considered as core competencies for each health profession. The literature strongly suggests that interprofessional competencies need to be part of the assessment framework for clinical education (Barr et al 2005, Davidson et al 2008). Explicit evaluation of interprofessional competencies as part of fieldwork assessment ensures that these competencies are valued in the same way as other assessed competencies and actively built into the learning objectives for a fieldwork placement. Students can see that interprofessional competencies are a core outcome of the fieldwork experience, potentially increasing the perceived relevance and importance of this skill set.

Build on existing programs, systems and interprofessional practice

Where effective interprofessional practice and clinical education already exist, they can be used as the springboard for increased *interprofessional* clinical education. Acknowledging and valuing areas where interprofessional practice and learning is already happening helps to build momentum for further expansion. Many health professionals already teach and promote interprofessional principles. With limited resources it makes sense to take advantage of any existing synchronicities in terms of timetabling, existing placement schedules, and available spaces and resources for collaborative learning.

As with student assessment, making interprofessional learning and practice explicit in departmental and organisational policy will foster a shift to seeing interprofessionalism as a core competency and value. This includes incorporating interprofessional approaches into performance management systems, position descriptions, appraisals, reward and recognition systems, and core institutional and departmental objectives.

What is the recipe?

There is no single recipe that describes how best to make interprofessional clinical education work. Perhaps in the end the set of guiding principles is the most appropriate framework for what is an extremely complex and dynamic activity. Although evidence is still emerging, we already have a considerable pool of knowledge about how to design, deliver and evaluate effective IPE programs. Most initiatives so far have been short-term pilot programs, so evaluation of longer term benefits to students and their future patients and clients has not yet been achieved.

Interprofessional education is a developing area in Australia. There is growing interest in implementing and evaluating interprofessional models of teaching—both within the university setting and in the fieldwork setting. Implementing IPE in the current intensified context of higher education and healthcare workplaces is a challenge not to be underestimated. It requires dedicated staff and substantial other resources over long periods of time. We have asserted in this chapter that change is needed on a number of levels to achieve this outcome: (1) policy and practice frameworks that endorse and promote the importance of interprofessional collaboration; and (2) further research to evaluate the effectiveness of interprofessional education in fostering interprofessional practice, and to demonstrate the impact that interprofessional practice has on patient outcomes, healthcare efficiency and effectiveness, and on staff recruitment, retention and satisfaction. We need to support a range of long-term, mixed-method research initiatives to establish the capacity of IPE to help improve IPP and then patient and client outcomes; (3) a reframing of interprofessional competency as a core competency for all healthcare professionals; (4) teaching approaches that emphasise the iterative development and application of interprofessional skills in practice; (5) collaborative approaches to teaching and learning; (6) shared language, labels and expectations for interprofessional approaches.

IPE needs to move from 'pilot project' to routine activity in Australia. Enabling health professionals to meet the future challenges of the healthcare system will require them to more effectively learn with, from, and about each other with the expressed purpose of improving collaboration and the quality of patient care.

References

Abdel-Halim RE 2006 Clinical methods and team work: 1,000 years ago. The American Journal of Surgery 191:289–290

ACT Health 2008 ACT Health Interprofessional Learning Project. Online. Available: http://health.act.gov.au/c/health?a=da&did=10153142 Accessed14 Jan 2009

Barr H 2002 Interprofessional education: today, yesterday and tomorrow: a review. Centre for the Advancement of Interprofessional Education (CAIPE), London

Barr H, Koppel I, Reeves S et al 2005 Effective interprofessional education: argument, assumption and evidence. Blackwell, Oxford

Braithwaite J, Travaglia JF 2005 Inter-professional learning and clinical education: an overview of the literature. Braithwaite & Associates & ACT Health Department

Curran V 2004 Interprofessional education for collaborative patient-centred practice research synthesis, Health Canada. Online. Available: http://www.hc-sc.gc.ca/hcs-sss/hhr-rhs/strateg/interprof/synth_e.html Accessed14 Jan 2009

Davidson M, Smith R, Dodd K et al 2008 Interprofessional clinical education: a systematic review. Australian Health Review 32(1):111–120

Day GE, Minichiello V, Madison J 2006 Nursing morale: what does the literature reveal? Australian Health Review 30(4):516–524

DeLoach R 2003 Job satisfaction among hospice interdisciplinary team members. American Journal of Hospice & Palliative Care 20(6):434–440

Department of Health 2001 Working together, learning together: a framework for lifelong learning of the NHS. Department of Health, London

Department of Human Services (DHS) 2007 Clinical placements in Victoria: establishing a statewide approach. Victorian Department of Human Services, Melbourne, Victoria

Ferrie J 2004 Work stress & health: the Whitehall II study. International Centre for Health and Society, Department of Epidemiology and Public Health, University College, London. Online. Available: http://www.ucl.ac.uk/whitehallII/findings/Whitehallbooklet.pdf Accessed 14 Jan 2009

Freeth D, Hammick M et al 2005 Effective interprofessional education: development, delivery and evaluation. Blackwell, Oxford

Graycar A 2008 Public policy: it's so obvious. ABC Radio National transcript from Ockham's Razor program. Online. Available: www.abc.net.au/rn/ockhamsrazor/stories/2008/2195706. htm#transcript Accessed 14 Jan 2009

Greene RJ, Cavell GF, Jackson SHD 1996 Interprofessional clinical education of medical and pharmacy students. Medical Education 30:129–133

Hackman JR, Oldham GR 1976 Motivation through the design of work. Organizational Behavior & Human Decision Processes 16(2):250–279

Herodotus 1954 The Histories. trans. Aubrey de Selincourt. Penguin, London

Illinois Institute of Technology 2008 Interprofessional projects program. Online. Available: http://ipro.iit.edu Accessed 14 Jan 2009

Karasek RA 1979 Job demands, job decision latitude, and mental strain: implications for job redesign. Administrative Science Quarterly 24:285–308

Kotter JP 1996 Leading change. Harvard Business School, Boston

Luecht RM, Madsen MK, Taugher MP, Petterson BJ 1990 Assessing professional perceptions: design and validation of an Interdisciplinary Education Perception Scale. Journal of Allied Health 19(2):181–191

McNair R, Stone N, Sims J, Curtis C 2005 Australian evidence for interprofessional education contributing to effective teamwork preparation and interest in rural practice. Journal of Interprofessional Care 19(6):579–594

Nair BR, Finucane PM 2003 Reforming medical education to enhance the management of chronic disease. Medical Journal of Australia 179(5):257–259

O'Halloran C, Hean S, Humphris D, Macleod-Clark J 2006 Developing common learning: the new generation project undergraduate curriculum model. Journal of Interprofessional Care 20(1):12–28

Reeves S, Freeth D 2002 The London training ward: an innovative interprofessional learning initiative. Journal of Interprofessional Care, 16(1):41–52

Reeves S, Zwarenstein M, Goldman J et al 2008 Interprofessional education: effects on professional practice and health care outcomes. Cochrane Database of Systematic Reviews, Issue 1, Art. No. CD002213. DOI: 10.1002/14651858.CD002213.pub2

Smith R, Watson L, Davidson M et al 2007 Learning together to work together: facilitating effective and cost-effective interprofessional clinical education—the Interprofessional Clinical Education (IPCE) project. Report to the Department of Human Services, Victoria. Online. Available: http://www.health.vic.gov.au/workforce/downloads/innovation.pdf Accessed15 Jan 2009

Snyder RC 1987 A societal backdrop for interprofessional education and practice. Theory into Practice 26(2):94–98

Stone N 2006a The Rural Interprofessional Education project. Journal of Interprofessional Care, 20(1):79–81

Stone N 2006b Evaluating interprofessional education: the tautological need for interdisciplinary approaches. Journal of Interprofessional Care 20(3):260–275

Stone N 2007 Coming in from the interprofessional cold in Australia. Australian Health Review 3(3):332–340

Stone N, Curtis C 2007 Interprofessional education in Victorian universities: key stakeholders' understandings, current practice, potential for expansion & context for change. Report funded by Department of Human Services, Victoria, Australia & School of Rural Health, University of Melbourne

World Health Organization (WHO) 1988 Learning together to work together for health. Report of a WHO study group on multiprofessional education for health personnel: the team approach. Technical Report Series 769:1–72, WHO, Geneva

Yan J, Gilbert JHV, Hoffman SJ 2007 Announcement. WHO Study group on interprofessional education and collaborative practice. Journal of Interprofessional Care 21(6):588–589

Zwarenstein M, Reeves S, Perrier L 2005 Effectiveness of pre-licensure interprofessional education and post-licensure collaborative interventions. Journal of Interprofessional Care 19:S148–S165

Recommended texts

Barr H, Koppel I, Reeves S et al 2005 Effective interprofessional education: argument, assumption and evidence. Blackwell, Oxford

Freeth D, Hammick M, Reeves S et al 2005 Effective interprofessional education: development, delivery and evaluation. Blackwell, Oxford

Websites

ACT Health Interprofessional Learning Project. Available: http://health.act.gov.au/ipl Accessed 14 Jan 2009

Center for Interprofessional Education (University of Minnesota). Available: www.ipe.umn.edu Accessed 14 Jan 2009

Canadian Interprofessional Health Initiative. Available: www.cihc.ca Accessed 14 Jan 2009

European Interprofessional Education Network. Available: http://www.eipen.org/ Accessed 14 Jan 2009

InterEd (The International Association for Interprofessional Education and Collaborative Practice). Available: http://www.interedhealth.org Accessed 14 Jan 2009

Interprofessional Network of British Columbia. Available: http://www.in-bc.ca/ Accessed 14 Jan 2009

New General Project, Universities of Southampton and Portsmouth. Available: http://www.commonlearning.net/default.htm Accessed 14 Jan 2009

Office of Interdisciplinary Health Sciences Education, East Carolina University. Available: http://www.ecu.edu/oihse/IRHTP.htm Accessed 14 Jan 2009

UK Centre for the Advancement of Interprofessional Education. Available: www.caipe.org.uk Accessed 14 Jan 2009

University of Sydney Interprofessional Learning Resources. Available: http://www.chs.usyd.edu.au/ipl/about/resources.php Accessed 14 Jan 2009

CHAPTER 6

Clinical education: embracing diversity

Anna Chur-Hansen and Robyn Woodward-Kron

THEORIES

In this chapter, medical anthropology provides the theoretical perspective to inform cultural representations of health, illness and healthcare practices. Applied linguistics and register theory provide a background framework to identify and analyse language and communication within student–patient and student–supervisor discourse.

USING THEORIES TO INFORM CURRICULUM DESIGN AND RESEARCH

Using the theoretical perspective of medical anthropology, explanatory models of health and illness and explanatory models of healthcare practice provide a practical means of highlighting and systematically incorporating different beliefs, values and experiences into the goals and structure of clinical education curricula. They provide a framework to assist students to recognise the impact of their own medical or healthcare models of practice and, importantly, a way to examine the patient's explanatory model of their illness. Using applied linguistics to analyse the structure of and meanings generated in clinical communication enables closer analysis of context, culture and expectations within the clinical communicative encounter.

USING THEORIES TO DRIVE EDUCATION METHODS

Having a theoretical understanding of the influence of diversity in both patients' and healthcare professionals' beliefs and value systems concerning illness and health can lead to specific teaching practices. These include expanding the types of questions that students use to elicit information from their patients, so that respect for the patient as an expert in their own health and illness is acknowledged. Including lectures that provide an anthropological perspective provide an additional source of information about the central values and philosophies that drive different healthcare practices. Teaching students how to analyse different aspects of their language during clinical interviews is a practical method that may increase levels of cultural competence in clinical communication.

Diversity in clinical education and healthcare provision

It is now recognised that health professional education and clinical practice encompass cultural variations both within and between professions, and between providers and recipients of care. Similarly students, practitioners, patients and clients represent a diversity of linguistic backgrounds. The assumed homogeneity of clinical education and healthcare provision is no longer an accepted construct. In Australia, overseas-born full-fee paying students and first-generation migrant school leavers are a well established presence in Australian medical schools (Hawthorne et al 2004) and in other health science disciplines (Hawthorne 2005a).

In clinical practice workforce shortages, particularly in rural areas, mean that overseas trained health professionals have come to play a critical role in healthcare provision and currently represent a substantial part of the healthcare workforce (Barton et al 2003, Birrell & Hawthorne 2004, Hawthorne 2005b). Furthermore, in migrant destination countries like Australia, diversity is not limited to the cultural diversity of the current and future healthcare workforce; cultural and linguistic diversity in the patient population is an integral component of the diversity landscape in clinical education and healthcare provision. Such diversity can pose substantial challenges for clinical educators and health professionals, and there is a small but growing literature on identifying and responding to these challenges.

Areas of concerns for students, international medical graduates (IMGs) and educators alike encompass communication skills and English language expertise in a range of domains, including using informal language appropriately (Chur-Hansen & Vernon-Roberts 1998, Hall et al 2004, Pilotto et al 2007, Saxena et al 2006, Woodward-Kron et al 2007a); the bio-psychosocial approach to patient-interviewing and the doctor–patient relationship (Haidet et al 2002, Liddell & Koritsas 2004); and the related issue of performance in examinations (Liddell & Koritsas 2004). It is worth noting that much of this literature is restricted to identifying difference and deficiency in performance of the overseas-born students and graduates in relation to dominant cultural norms, desired behaviours and practices. For example, differences include overseas-born students' reported preference for a bio-medical model of patient interviewing rather than a bio-psychosocial one (Liddell & Koritsas 2004), while deficiencies are evident in students' lack of sufficient local cultural and linguistic knowledge to establish rapport and ask more sensitive questions when interviewing patients (Chur-Hansen & Vernon-Roberts 1998).

While acknowledging the very real challenges these issues present to clinical educators and learners, this chapter aims to extend current awareness about cultural diversity in clinical education to include diversity as a potential learning and teaching resource. The chapter argues that an interdisciplinary approach, drawing on the fields of medical anthropology and applied linguistics respectively, can better equip clinical educators to meet the needs of culturally heterogeneous students and patients. It examines notions of cultural competence and models of health and illness in order to challenge our own culturally informed perspectives and regulated behaviours, which inform our clinical practice and decision making. It also introduces a model of language in context in order to better conceptualise the contextual variables crucial to effective intercultural communication.

Notions of cultural competence
Culture and the notion of cultural competence

There is a tendency in clinical practice to imagine that 'culture' is a concept that separates 'us' from 'them'. That is, we tend to understand culture as a construct that explains differences between two groups. In Australia the groupings most commonly recognised are 'us', 'Westerners', who are different from 'them', meaning anyone else who does not fit into this dominant cultural category. A secondary grouping that is also considered is that of 'us' as healthcare professionals, placed in juxtaposition to 'them', those who are patients or clients (Tilburt & Geller 2007). This latter distinction is often implicit—clinical reality is rarely explicitly discussed as a cultural construct, nor is it often acknowledged that the biomedical approach is culture specific and value laden (Kleinman et al 1978, Hahn & Kleinman 1983).

To understand culture as a dichotomy in this way is simplistic and misleading. Everyone lives within and is a product of 'culture'. In simple terms, culture refers to a system of ideas and beliefs, including values and ideals, which are held in common by a community of people with a system of shared meanings (Chur-Hansen et al 2006). Culture is heterogeneous: an individual functions within and is shaped by a number of subcultural identities. For example, gender, sexuality, religion and religiosity, marital status, age, level of education and employment (or lack of employment) are all examples of subcultural groupings. Within these subcultures, while common ideas and beliefs will be apparent, there will be individual variations. Similarly, in the healthcare professions, while the biomedical model could be arguably seen as the dominant cultural framework, there are a number of differences in understanding and approach, both within medicine and its various specialities, and between and within the different healthcare professions themselves, such as dentistry, medicine, nursing, physiotherapy and psychology. In addition, existing alongside recognised Western healthcare professions are those practitioners who also contribute to subcultural understandings about illness and disease, and offer treatment including, for example, traditional healers, religious leaders and alternative and complementary medicine providers.

With complexities around cultural and subcultural differences in communities, along with differences on an individual level, health professional students and practising clinicians are faced with a complex challenge. It is not appropriate to assume that dominant cultural categories (such as 'Western' and 'biomedical model' approaches to healthcare) must take priority, and that therefore proficiency in these will be sufficient. To operate on this level is ethnocentric, or as Kleinman et al (1978 p 251) term it, 'medicocentric'— the belief that one's own cultural understandings are superior to all others (Keesing & Strathern 1998). However, it is also unrealistic to imagine that any one person can have a working knowledge and understanding of every possible cultural and subcultural perspective. Clinicians and undergraduate students and trainees need to demonstrate an ability to work with people from a variety of different backgrounds, including eliciting their narratives about what they think is wrong and what they think needs to happen next. Thus healthcare practitioners need to demonstrate 'cultural competence', which has been defined by Anderson et al (2003) as including the capacity to identify, understand, and respect the values and beliefs of others (p 74). More specifically, Carpenter-Song et al (2007) explain cultural competence as the application of specific techniques and skills by an individual in the context of clinical encounters, and the promotion of organisational practices to meet the needs of diverse populations (p 1363).

There are a number of models of cultural competency for training healthcare professionals. Carpenter-Song et al (2007) have summarised the shortcomings identified by medical anthropologists who have critiqued these models. Criticisms include presenting culture as static; treating culture as a variable; conflating culture with race and ethnicity; failing to acknowledge diversity within groups; inadvertently placing blame on a patient's culture; emphasising cultural differences and thereby obscuring structural power imbalances; and finally, failing to recognise biomedicine as a cultural system itself (p 1363). In addition to addressing these concerns in any cultural competency model, the premise of medical anthropologists is that biomedical culture must be modified to be culturally appropriate to the patient, and that it is this approach that can facilitate the cultural competency of practitioners (Dein 2004).

Explanatory models of illness

Arthur Kleinman is Professor of Medical Anthropology in Social Medicine and Professor of Psychiatry, Harvard Medical School (Online. Available: http//www.fas.harvard.edu/9 Jan 2009). His seminal work in medical anthropology on explanatory models has been influential in medical education (in behavioural sciences curricula) and in the training and clinical practice of psychiatrists. First published in the 1970s, it is only recently that other health professional training programs have incorporated this concept into curricula or clinical practice. There is very little in the published literature about explanatory models outside of medicine. However, for an example in dentistry see Nations and de Araujo Soares Nuto (2002), in epidemiology see Weiss (2001), in nursing see McSweeny et al (1997), and in physiotherapy see Hunt (2007).

Kleinman and his colleagues (Kleinman et al 1978, Kleinman 1980, 1988a, 1988b) note that patient and clinician explanatory models share five common issues: aetiology, onset of symptoms, pathophysiology, course of illness (including type of sick role—acute, chronic, impaired—and severity of disorder), and treatment. Patient explanatory models reflect social class, cultural beliefs, education, occupation, religious affiliation and past experiences with illness and with healthcare. Kleinman et al (1978, p 256) state:

> Eliciting the patient model gives the physician knowledge of the beliefs the patient holds about his illness, the personal and social meaning he attaches to his disorder, his expectations about what will happen to him and what the doctor will do, and his own therapeutic goals. Comparison of patient model with the doctor's model enables the clinician to identify major discrepancies that may cause problems in clinical management. Such comparisons also help the clinician know which aspects of his explanatory model need clearer exposition to patients (and families), and what sort of patient education is most appropriate. And they clarify conflicts not related to different levels of knowledge but different values and interests. Part of the clinical process involves negotiations between these explanatory models, once they have been made explicit.

To utilise the explanatory model concept in clinical practice it is necessary to elicit the patient's explanatory model in a systematic way, showing genuine interest and respect. The patient is the expert as it is they who are experiencing this illness, and thus they are asked to explain what is happening, from their perspective, to the healthcare practitioner.

Kleinman et al (1978) suggest the following questions: (1) What do you think has caused your problem?; (2) Why do you think it started when it did?; (3) What do you think your sickness does to you? How does it work?; (4) How severe is your sickness? Will it have a short or long course?; (5) What kind of treatment do you think you should receive?; (6) What are the most important results you hope to receive from this treatment?; (7) What are the chief problems your sickness has caused for you?; (8) What do you fear most about your sickness? (p 256).

In negotiations between the patient and the healthcare professional's explanatory model, discrepancies are identified and discussed. Some discrepancies can be recognised but need not be changed, for example, if a person is willing to take medication but also wishes to consult a fortune-teller, the healthcare professional should respect this. Where the patient is unwilling to accept the biomedical treatment for their problem, the healthcare professional needs to negotiate, to try and find a mutually agreeable compromise. Kleinman et al (1978) consider the negotiation stage to be perhaps the single most important step in building trust, promoting adherence and increasing patient satisfaction. On a practitioner level, this process can be seen as facilitating reflexive practice, a personal and professional quality that is valued in current health professional education pedagogy (Tilburt & Geller 2007).

The concept of explanatory models of illness and their role in cultural competency has been applauded because it is practically relevant; it is not simply a theory (Phillips 1985). Furthermore, the concept is able to manage the physical reductionism and Cartesianism of biomedicine: the explanatory model concept does this, as it juxtaposes the medical model with the patient's—both are considered valid (Phillips 1985). It addresses the concerns outlined by Carpenter-Song et al (2007). That is, it can accommodate change over time, take into account irrational beliefs and hidden meanings, accept diversity between and among groups, because in the clinical setting it focuses on the individual rather than any one particular group, and recognises that the healthcare professions are a culture unto themselves and this must be taken into account in clinical practice (Kleinman 1981). Discussing explanatory models facilitates communication, and this, it has been proposed, is instrumental in improving disparities in healthcare (Ashton et al 2003).

However, while it is generally accepted that the explanatory model concept is a useful one in the demonstration of cultural competence, there are some limitations to its use that have been discussed in the literature. It has been argued that people's explanatory models can be vague, have multiple levels of meaning, change frequently, and blur ideas and experience (Rajaram & Rashidi 1998). Eliciting and understanding them may not be straightforward. It has also been noted that explanatory models are fluid (Williams & Healy 2001), dynamic, and evolve over time as contact with biomedicine influences affects understandings of illness (Schreiber & Hartrick 2002). Thus the explanatory model offered by a particular patient at one time may not be the same one offered at a later date. This is not necessarily problematic, as long as the healthcare practitioner is cognisant of this, and reviews the patient's explanatory models accordingly. Williams and Healy (2001) suggest that explanatory models might be more properly called 'explanatory maps' to reflect their unstable nature. McSweeny et al (1997), from the perspective of nursing research and practice, document several limitations to the approach. They call for more research into the utility of using the concept of explanatory models for improving patient outcomes, as to date there is a dearth of evidence to show that cultural competency training of any type has an impact on health outcomes, a point also made by Betancourt (2003).

In a review of culturally competent healthcare systems, including a review of cultural competency training for healthcare providers by Anderson et al (2003), the efficacy of training could not be reported because so few studies have evaluated outcomes pre- and post-training, or compared different training interventions. The issue of the amount of time needed to elicit and explore a person's explanatory model in the clinical setting has also been underscored by McSweeny et al (1997): they suggest the approach is possibly more advantageous when multiple encounters with a patient are feasible. Additional time facilitates trust and rapport, so the individual is more comfortable in disclosing their thoughts about their illness. Lloyd et al (1998) have developed a Short Explanatory Model Interview (SEMI), which is brief, standardised and validated, in an attempt to address the issue of time limitations, particularly where the elicitation of the explanatory model from a group of patients is undertaken for the purpose of research. McSweeny et al (1997) further note that the negotiation phase between the patient and healthcare professional's explanatory models assumes an equality of power that rarely exists, and with which the patient might not be comfortable, if the negotiation phase were offered. This is an issue which needs to be considered on a case-by-case basis, and will in itself require a level of cultural competency in making a judgement about the patient's preferred role in the clinical encounter. An important point to be made about the use of explanatory models in clinical practice is that elicitation, understanding and negotiation all require considerable skill on the part of the clinician, and these skills must be taught. We therefore turn our attention to the concept of explanatory models and cultural competency training in health professional curricula.

Explanatory models and cultural competency training in health professional curricula

Carrese and Marshall (2000) note that calls have been made for anthropology to be taught to medical students and trainees since 1892. Yet to date, medical anthropology is not usually considered core curriculum in most medical schools, although there is usually some limited anthropological content. It is certainly not core, or perhaps even viewed as relevant, in all health professional curricula. In medical schools and postgraduate medicine training programs, cultural competence training seems to be limited to single lectures or workshops, rather than being part of an integrated, core curriculum (Kripalani et al 2006). In 1985 Phillips warned that to survive as a discipline, medical anthropology must be viewed as fundamental to medical practice, rather than seen as dispensable in times of financial pressure or with competing demands on curricula time: this remains a continuing challenge.

Several authors have outlined ways in which cultural competency training might be incorporated into core curriculum. They write from the perspective of medical education. However, the principles can be readily applied across broader health professional education.

In a collected volume edited by Chrisman and Maretzki (1982), six chapters are devoted to the teaching of clinically applied anthropology, four of them focusing on medicine, but one dealing with nursing (Chrisman 1982) and another with nutrition and food science (Ritenbaugh 1982). While dated, this volume is recommended as a valuable resource for the educator interested in designing cultural competency training for health professional students. Kripalani et al (2006) reviewed more current approaches to cultural competency training and propose factors that should be considered in designing any curriculum. They see the explanatory model approach as one that allows transferable skills to be developed, rather than simply imparting knowledge-based information that cannot be readily applied; a point made clearly by Kleinman and his colleagues when first proposing the utility of the concept. Betancourt (2003) agrees that applied skills are necessary in training, but cautions that training in cultural knowledge and attitudes should also be fundamental to any cultural competency training. Interactive educational methods are considered preferable to passive learning techniques. These include standardised patient encounters (Carrillo et al 1999), role-plays and reflective journals.[1]

Feedback for students and trainees from teachers who have had cultural competence training and have used culturally appropriate strategies in their own clinical work, is more desirable than teaching from educators who are speaking in theoretical terms only. Finally, it is widely agreed that cultural competence should be integrated throughout the curriculum, rather than comprising a one-off workshop or an isolated lecture or two (Kripalani et al 2006, Carrese & Marshall 2000, Phillips 1985).

There is a major gap in the health professional education research literature, and this needs to be considered when designing cultural competency curricula. Kripalani et al (2006) recommend that students are shown evidence for why culture is important in healthcare and how cultural competence training is valuable. However, they acknowledge, as have others (Thom et al 2006, Anderson et al 2003, Betancourt 2003) that educators will need to draw on very limited research. Thus it is important that cultural competence training has an evaluative component, for example, pre- and post-testing, Objective Structured Clinical Examinations (OSCEs) and video-taped clinical encounters for rating and reviewing.

Educators need to collect data in a systematic and rigorous manner to provide an evidence base and inform future curricula design. Betancourt (2003) discusses three important challenges to evaluating the efficacy of cultural competency training interventions. Social desirability response bias means that true attitudes, perceptions and reactions may not be captured, and thus the validity of collected data is an issue. In addition, assessing knowledge via testing 'facts' about culture may inadvertently lead to encouraging stereotyping and, furthermore, does not mean that this knowledge translates into practice. Also, evaluations from students and trainees regarding cultural competencies and training may reflect a perception that the material is 'soft', and thus reactions and evaluations may be skewed in a negative direction. For these reasons, Betancourt recommends a mixed-methods evaluative approach, including surveys, pre- and post-testing of knowledge and attitudes, and presentation of clinical cases and OSCES. It would be useful to add a qualitative component through interviewing stakeholders (students, teachers, clinicians, clients and patients, curriculum designers and so forth) to supplement any quantitative measures. These mixed methodologies may help us to understand the short- and medium-term impact of training on cultural competencies, and how to improve training interventions and curriculum design. As already discussed, the longer term influence of training on patient or client health outcomes, along with the effect cultural competence has upon the practitioner in terms of work satisfaction for instance, is yet to be carefully studied.

Intercultural clinical communication

Expectations and assumptions about the manner in which a consultation in a healthcare setting should unfold, the type and range of questions the health professional should ask, and the desired and perceived outcomes of a consultation are influenced by cultural background. Important aspects of the consultation needing to be considered are that of spoken and non-verbal language.

....
1 For an explanation and overview of the standardised patient approach in health professional education the reader is referred to Chur-Hansen and Burg (2006).

In healthcare provision, language plays a crucial role in bridging cultural differences: in establishing rapport and trust so that necessary information can be elicited; in providing information and advice to patients that is acceptable to both the patients' health beliefs and practices as well as to the healthcare provider; in treatment decision making and so on. Language proficiency in healthcare is more than a high degree of spoken, non-verbal and written fluency in health professional discourses (e.g. interacting efficiently in multidisciplinary teams, with patients, with colleagues and so on): it includes the capability to interact effectively with patients in terms of the larger cultural context in which the health professional is practising. This involves interacting with the varieties of the dominant language present in the particular context; for example, in Australia this includes Australian English, Singaporean English ('Singlish'), Malaysian English, Koori English, Italo–Australian English, and Greek Australian English, as well as the varieties within those dialects (rural and urban variation, generational variation, socioeconomic variation and so on). It also involves being responsive to the culturally determined beliefs and attitudes of those particular subgroups.

As previously mentioned, much of the literature on communication skills of overseas-born students and graduates focuses on difference and deficiency from the perspective of clinical supervisors. In order to better understand the challenges of intercultural clinical communication, the perspectives of overseas-born students and graduates can be useful to identify areas of cultural dissonance and knowledge gaps that may not be apparent to clinical educators, particularly if they share the same cultural background as the dominant culture. Furthermore, other disciplinary perspectives can provide new approaches and frameworks for teaching and learning clinical communication. The next section reports on an Australian study investigating overseas-born students' perspectives of the cultural and linguistic challenges of clinical communication. It includes a linguistic perspective of the challenges of student–patient interviewing for overseas-born students.

Overseas-born student perspectives of intercultural clinical communication

Thirty-one overseas-born students from a range of cultural backgrounds and three health science disciplines (medicine, physiotherapy and nursing) participated in individual and focus group interviews to identify, from their point of view, the main cultural and linguistic differences and challenges they had encountered during their clinical placements (Woodward-Kron et al 2007a). The study was conducted by University of Melbourne academics from the Faculty of Medicine, Dentistry and Health Sciences' International Student Support Program, an embedded program providing academic and professional English support to the faculty's large number of overseas-born students. The motivation for the study for the researchers was to extend their knowledge gained through observation and experience of the students' learning needs, and to inform the design and delivery of support communication workshops. It also informed the development of a multimedia DVD-ROM on intercultural clinical communication.

The findings showed that the students who participated in the interviews were well aware of cultural differences in the clinical settings, as well as how culture impacted on how they interacted with patients. It is worth noting that in the students' responses, more comments were made about cultural differences and how this impacted on communication than on their language proficiency per se, underscoring the important role of culture in communication. Themes which emerged from the interviews were the greater emphasis on patient-centredness in Australia compared to students' home environments, the greater degree of patient autonomy as well as Australian patients' greater knowledge about their own health, and health prevention measures and treatment options.

Despite the cultural diversity of the participants in the study, a recurring and dominant finding was the perception of the pervasiveness of alcohol in Australian society, with most respondents referring to the ubiquity of alcohol and drinking. Participants demonstrated awareness that they needed to remain non-judgemental when speaking to patients about alcohol consumption, and several commented on their lack of knowledge about alcohol and Australian socially acceptable drinking practices.

Other behavioural differences included the observation by several African and Asian students on the relationships between different generations in Australian families as well as differences in the degree of respect and obedience shown to elders. Students particularly identified that the need to show respect to older generations in their cultures made it challenging for them to ask personal and sensitive questions of older adults in the Australian setting.

Numerous participants demonstrated awareness of informal language for establishing rapport and putting patients at ease, and most were aware that they needed to increase their knowledge of slang and colloquial terms so that they knew which words were taboo and which were acceptable, particularly for talking about bodily functions.

The students' perspectives elicited in this study provide culturally influenced explanations of and background information to their possible problems with aspects of student–patient interviewing which may impact on their performance. The findings can also inform clinical educators and locally born students on communicating with culturally diverse patients because as yet few studies (e.g. Chur-Hansen 1999) address any potential interconnections between intercultural communication issues for undergraduate and graduate students and patient cultural diversity.

A linguistic perspective of the challenges of student–patient interviewing for overseas-born students

The findings from the overseas-born students' perspectives of clinical communication study informed the development of a DVD-ROM on clinical communication for overseas-born students (Woodward-Kron et al 2007b). The DVD-ROM includes four student–patient scenarios which incorporate aspects of communication challenges identified in the students' perspectives study: these were an alcohol history taking, a social history taking, paediatric asthma management, and chronic pain management. These semi-scripted student–patient interviews were designed as triggers for reflecting on and practising a number of communication requirements, strategies and skills. The student participants in the videos were overseas-born students in the faculty who had a high level of communication skills, including fluency; however the final videos include minor hesitations, misunderstandings, grammatical inaccuracies, and some awkwardness in manner. These aspects informed the content of some of the reflection tasks. Despite the semi-scripted nature of the interviews, a number of communication challenges and areas for development occurred, challenges primarily relating to language use in particular contexts. These can be summarised as follows:

- student unfamiliarity with informal and colloquial language used by the patient, for example, 'What's a G and T (gin and tonic)?'

- student unfamiliarity and comprehension problems with jokes made by the patient
- student awkwardness when attempting to elicit information on family relationships and sensitive related psycho-social aspects, resulting in breaks in the flow of conversation and partial confusion for the patient
- extensive and at times excessive use of politeness markers by the student when eliciting information
- student hesitancy when probing about psycho-social aspects; this contributed to patient unease about the direction of the interview
- a limited repertoire of student responses to show empathy and build rapport, for example, student participants relied heavily on the formulaic 'that must be hard for you' to show empathy
- a limited repertoire of initiating open questions to maintain the flow of the interview, for example, one participant relied on 'how about' to open up new directions of enquiry, that is, 'How about your work?', 'How about your boyfriend?' resulting in considerable repetition
- student lack of conversational and signposting strategies as well as confidence when signalling a more sensitive area of enquiry, for example, 'I'd just like to ask you a few questions about your diet and everything'.

The communication problems and infelicities noted above can be partly attributed to the intersection of language and culture in the context of the student–patient interview, although it should be understood that some of these weaknesses in interview technique are common to all novice students. The causes of these infelicities and communication 'sticking points' can be classified into three broad areas (Woodward-Kron 2008). The first of these is to do with the 'what' of the interaction, that is, what the participants are talking about. This includes the colloquial language used to refer to items, processes and practices possibly outside the students' experiences. The second is to do with the 'who' of the interaction—the impact of status, age, experience, role and so on in the interaction. The third is to do with the 'how' of the interaction, that is, how the interaction unfolds and progresses.

A model for relating context and language in the student–patient interview

These contextual aspects of the student–patient interview, the 'what', 'who', and 'how', and how this is realised in language reflect the intersection of the broader context of student cultural backgrounds, local culture and language varieties, and the culture and language of patient interviewing. In order to examine the intercultural dimension of student–patient interviewing and to support students in developing their communication skills, a model of language in context from the field of applied linguistics can assist in systematically addressing these areas of concern. This has been elaborated in Woodward-Kron (2008) and a synopsis is provided below.

Much of the work of the linguist Michael Halliday has been concerned with how people use language in context to get things done. Halliday's (1979) model relating language and context, which is referred to as register theory, is informed by the work of the anthropologist Malinowski. The model incorporates two levels of context: the immediate environment of communication, which is referred to as *the context of situation*, and the broader surrounding environment, referred to as *the context of culture*. For communication to occur, Halliday (1979, Halliday & Hasan 1985) argues that it is necessary for those who are participating in the interaction to be able to make informed guesses about what kinds of meanings (and language) are likely to be exchanged. As participants, we make predictions about the types of meanings that will be exchanged based on the immediate context of the situation. Students and patients can predict aspects of the interview as it unfolds: for example, the types of questions that will be asked and to some extent the words used. The broader cultural context in which the interview occurs allows students to predict other aspects, such as the degree of formality expected or the necessary psycho-social background questions, and the public health concerns which should be raised (e.g. regular screening, diet, exercise, smoking and alcohol intake). In order to distinguish and interpret the social contexts of texts, register theory identifies three variables, namely, field, tenor and mode. Field refers to what is happening or the content dimension of the text; tenor refers to the roles and role relationships of the participants in the text; while mode refers to what part language is playing, including the organisation of the text, and how it unfolds (Halliday & Hasan 1985, p 12).

Table 6.1 maps register theory onto aspects of student–patient interviewing, identifying some of the possible contextual factors and meanings. The column identifying intercultural aspects includes possible areas of concern from an intercultural clinical communication perspective as reflected in the previous section. The intercultural aspects reflect the context of culture, while the student–patient interview column reflects the more immediate context of situation.

REGISTER VARIABLES	STUDENT–PATIENT INTERVIEW	INTERCULTURAL ASPECTS
FIELD of the discourse—content	• medical terminology for illness and symptoms as well as everyday language • family relations, job, lifestyle–emotional well-being, institutions • narration of course of illness or relevant events	• colloquial language for illness and symptoms • knowledge of institutions and cultural norms
TENOR of the discourse—role relations	• student–learner health professional and patient (age and sociocultural background, expertise) • affective involvement (positive or negative) • degree of familiarity–formality	• behaviours and practices • family relations and structure • conversational dimension and affective responses • respect for age and/or status
MODE of the discourse—role of language	• topic shifts, from medical to interpersonal dimension • dialogue or interactive discussion with negotiation and/or dynamic exchanges • temporal sequencing, course of illness or events • causes, elicitation of cause of illness, concerns, feelings	• flow of the interaction, cohesion • relevant topic shifts • clarification

Table 6.1 A register perspective of the intercultural student–patient interview (adapted from Woodward-Kron 2008)

The framework of the register variables field, tenor and mode has the potential to be used as an analytical tool to conceptualise the student–patient interview within its immediate context of situation as well as within the broader context of culture. As it is presented here, it requires little specialist knowledge of language to be used by health professional educators with students.

While the emphasis in this chapter has been on the communication needs of overseas-born students, the predictive capacity of the framework means that it can be used with both locally born and overseas-born students to elicit the types of meaning which could occur in a particular health provision scenario in a given context or situation, while taking into account the broader context of culture. Both local and overseas-born students can act as informants about cultural aspects, behaviours, expectations for the 'tenor' (interpersonal) dimension, while local students can assist with building their overseas-born colleagues' knowledge of colloquial language and the contexts in which it can be appropriately used. In addition to the predictive dimension of the model, it has the capacity to be used as a feedback device when students practise their interviewing skills in role-play scenarios or with a simulated patient. It would allow systematic feedback to be given on positive as well as negative aspects of student interview performance from the perspective of content (field), relationship–rapport–patient-centredness (tenor), and flow–cohesion detail of presenting problem (mode). The register model of language in context can supplement existing detailed assessment protocols or can be used by students as a simple but systematic tool to provide feedback to colleagues on various aspects of their performance.

While not elaborated in this chapter, Halliday's model of language in context is related to another more detailed model of language that provides an overview of the language choices (the lexicogrammar or the words and grammatical structures) available to the participants for the three areas of the model. Explanation of this more detailed model is beyond the scope of this chapter; suffice to say that for language specialists providing academic and professional English support to overseas-born students, it allows more detailed and systematic language work to be done which is sensitive to both the immediate context of situation (the student–patient interview) as well as to the broader context of culture (in this instance, Western educational and cultural values, culturally diverse patients and students).

Conclusion

Previous authors have approached cultural competency and the role of language background in the clinical encounter from a model that assumes the medical model and speakers of English as a first language to be 'gold standard'. The implicit assumption from this approach is that non-medical and non-Western conceptualisations of health and illness are interesting or curious, but invalid. Similarly, students, healthcare professionals and patients from language backgrounds other than English are seen to have problems that need to be addressed, working on a model of 'remediation' or deficit (J Crichton & K Lushington, unpublished).

In this chapter we have argued that there has always been cultural and linguistic diversity in the healthcare professions. Dentistry, medicine, nursing, occupational therapy, physiotherapy, psychology or any of the other health professions have never been homogeneous, despite being presented as such. By making this notion explicit, pedagogical and research approaches can be utilised that recognise not only diversity, but also the ethnocentrism of assuming that one approach or one language background is superior to any other. Rather than looking for ways to force behaviours into a standardised world view, future educators and researchers need to consider how to draw upon the wealth of difference available and the opportunities arising as a consequence for learning from others.

We have argued that the concepts of explanatory models and register theory are valuable in embracing differences in culture and language background, and can be readily incorporated into clinical teaching strategies. We have also argued that drawing upon different disciplines, and in particular cultural anthropology, can help clinical educators to develop new ways of thinking about the strengths that the heterogeneity of students, practitioners, clients and patients have to offer.

References

Anderson LM, Scrimshaw SC, Fullilove MT et al 2003 Culturally competent health care systems. American Journal of Preventive Medicine 24:68–79

Ashton CM, Haidet P, Paterniti DA et al 2003 Racial and ethnic disparities in the use of health services. Bias, preferences or poor communication? Journal of General Internal Medicine 18:146–152

Barton D, Hawthorne L, Singh B et al 2003 Victoria's dependence on overseas trained doctors in psychiatry. People and Place 11(1):54–64

Betancourt JR 2003 Cross-cultural medical education: conceptual approaches and frameworks for evaluation. Academic Medicine 78: 560–569

Birrell B, Hawthorne L 2004 Medicare plus and overseas-trained medical doctors. People and Place 12(2):83–99

Carrese JA, Marshall PA 2000 Teaching anthropology in the medical curriculum. Southern Society for Clinical Investigation 319:297–305

Carpenter-Song EA, Nordquest Schwallie M, Longhofer J 2007 Cultural competence re-examined: critique and directions for the future. Psychiatric Services 58:1362–1365

Carrillo JE, Green AR, Betancourt JR 1999 Cross-cultural primary care: a patient-based approach. Annals of Internal Medicine 130:829–834

Chrisman NJ 1982 Anthropology in Nursing: An exploration of adaptation. In: Chrisman NJ, Maretzki TW (eds) Clinically applied anthropology. D Reidel, Dordrecht, 117–140

Chrisman NJ, Maretzki TW (eds) 1982 Clinically applied anthropology. D Reidel, Dordrecht

Chur-Hansen A 1999 Teaching support in the behavioural sciences for non-English speaking background medical undergraduates. Medical Education 33:404–410

Chur-Hansen A, Burg FD 2006 Working with standardised patients for teaching and learning. The Clinical Teacher 3:220–224

Chur-Hansen A, Caruso J, Sumpowthong K et al 2006 Cross-cultural and Indigenous issues in psychology. Pearson Education, Frenchs Forest, NSW

Chur-Hansen A, Vernon-Roberts J 1998 Clinical teachers' perceptions of medical students' English language proficiency. Medical Education 32:351–356

Dein S 2004 Explanatory models of and attitudes towards cancer in different cultures. Lancet Oncology 5:119–124

Hahn RA, Kleinman A 1983 Biomedical practice and anthropological theory: frameworks and directions. Annual Review of Anthropology 12:305–333

Haidet P, Dains J, Paterniti D et al 2002 Medical student attitudes towards the doctor–patient relationship. Medical Education 36:568–574

Hall P, Keely E, Dojeiji S et al 2004 Communication skills, cultural challenges and individual support: challenges of international medical graduates in a Canadian healthcare environment. Medical Teacher 26(2):120–125

Halliday MAK 1979 Modes of meaning and modes of expression: types of grammatical structure and their determination by different semantic functions. In: Allerton D, Carney E, Hollcroft D (eds) Functions and context in linguistic analysis: a Festschrift for William Haas. Cambridge University Press, UK, p 57–79

Halliday MAK, Hasan R 1985 Language, context and text: aspects of language in a social-semiotic perspective. Deakin University Press, Geelong, Victoria

Hawthorne L 2005a Faculty internationalisation issues paper 28: National student demand for Australian health science courses. Faculty of Medicine, Dentistry and Health Sciences, University of Melbourne

Hawthorne L 2005b Picking winners: the recent transformation of Australia's skill migration policy. International Migration review 39:663–696

Hawthorne L, Minas H, Singh B 2004 A case study in the globalisation of medical education: assisting overseas-born students at the University of Melbourne. Medical Teacher 26:150–159

Hunt M 2007 Taking culture seriously: considerations for physiotherapists. Physiotherapy 93:229–232

Keesing RM, Strathern AJ 1998 Cultural anthropology: a contemporary perspective, 3rd edn. Harcourt Brace, Fort Worth

Kleinman A 1980 Patients and healers in the context of culture. An exploration of the borderland between anthropology, medicine and psychiatry. University of California Press, Berkeley

Kleinman A 1981 On illness meanings and clinical interpretation: not 'rational man', but a rational approach to man the sufferer/man the healer. Culture, Medicine and Psychiatry 5: 373–377

Kleinman A 1988a Rethinking psychiatry: from cultural category to personal experience. Free Press, New York

Kleinman A 1988b The illness narratives: suffering, healing and the human condition. Basic Books, New York

Kleinman A, Eisenberg L, Good B 1978 Clinical lessons from anthropologic and cross-cultural research. Annals of Internal Medicine 88:251–258

Kripalani S, Bussey-Jones J, Katz MG et al 2006 A prescription for cultural competence in medical education. Journal of General Internal Medicine 21:1116–1120

Liddell M, Koritsas S 2004 Effect of medical students' ethnicity on their attitudes towards consultation skills and final year examination performance. Medical Education 38:187–198

Lloyd KR, Jacob KS, Patel V et al 1998 The development of the Short Explanatory Model Interview (SEMI) and its use among primary-care attenders with common mental disorders. Psychological Medicine 28:1231–1237

McSweeney JC, Allan JD, Mayo K 1997 Exploring the use of explanatory models in nursing research and practice. Journal of Nursing Scholarship 29:243–248

Nations MK, de Araujo Soares Nuto S 2002 'Tooth worms', poverty tattoos and dental care conflicts in North-east Brazil. Social Science and Medicine 54:229–244

Phillips MR 1985 Can 'Clinically Applied Anthropology' survive in medical care settings? Medical Anthropology Quarterly 16:31–36

Pilotto L, Duncan G, Anderson-Wurf J 2007 Issues for clinicians training international medical graduates. Medical Journal of Australia 187:225–228

Rajaram SS, Rashidi A 1998 Minority women and breast cancer screening: the role of cultural explanatory models. Preventative Medicine 27:757–764

Ritenbaugh C 1982 New approaches to old problems: interactions of culture and nutrition. In: Chrisman NJ, Maretzki TW (eds) Clinically applied anthropology. D Reidel, Dordrecht, p 141–178

Saxena S, Dennis S, Vagholkar S et al 2006 Assessment of the learning needs of international medical graduates. Focus on Health Professional Education 8:49–57

Schreiber R, Hartrick G 2002 Keeping it together: how women use the biomedical explanatory model to manage the stigma of depression. Issues in Mental Health Nursing 23: 91–105

Thom DH, Tirado MD, Wood TL et al 2006 Development and evaluation of a cultural competency training curriculum. BMC Medical Education 6:38 doi:10.1186/1472–6920–6–38

Tilburt J, Geller G 2007 The importance of Worldviews for Medical Education. Academic Medicine 82: 819–822

Weiss MG 2001 Cultural epidemiology: an introduction and overview. Anthropology and Medicine 8:5–29

Williams B, Healy D 2001 Perceptions of illness causation among new referrals to a community mental health team: 'explanatory model' or 'explanatory map'? Social Science and Medicine 53:465–476

Woodward-Kron R 2008 Learner medical discourse and intercultural clinical communication: towards a contextually informed teaching framework. In: Solly M (ed.) Verbal/Visual narrative texts in higher education. Peter Lang, Linguistics Insights Series, Zurich, p 279–298

Woodward-Kron R, Hamilton J, Rischin I 2007a Managing cultural differences, diversity and the dodgy: overseas-born students' perspectives of clinical communication in Australia. Focus on Health Professional Education 9(3):30–43

Woodward-Kron R, Hamilton J, Rischin I et al 2007b 'I'm feeling a bit crook': understanding and managing clinical communication in Australia. DVD-ROM, University of Melbourne

Acknowledgements

Anna Chur-Hansen is indebted to the late Professor Rob Barrett, who first introduced her to the concept of explanatory models in medical anthropology and their application in clinical health professional education, particularly their utility in medical and psychiatric education.

Material in this chapter was presented by Dr Chur-Hansen at the Intercultural Clinical Communication in Health Professional Education Symposium, University of Melbourne, Australia, 8 February 2008.

Section 3

Applying knowledge: teaching and learning practices

CHAPTER 7

Clinical reasoning: the nuts and bolts of clinical education

Rola Ajjawi, Stephen Loftus, Henk G Schmidt and Silvia Mamede

THEORIES

Two theoretical perspectives are highlighted in this chapter. *Cognitive psychology* and *behaviourism* provide the theoretical bases for the analysis of the steps involved in processing information in clinical reasoning. A cognitively based understanding of the way clinicians make sense of clinical presentations assists in distinguishing between clinical reasoning in experts and novices. *Interpretivisim* is a social sciences theory that emphasises different understandings of an experience or phenomenon. Using interpretivism as a frame of reference for clinical reasoning means attention is paid to the social world of people, their stories and relevant policies, institutions and cultures.

USING THEORIES TO INFORM CURRICULUM DESIGN AND RESEARCH

When designing clinical education curricula to foster clinical reasoning, educators need to include learning tasks that incorporate the cognitively based hypothetico-deductive processes involved, in addition to broader sociocultural influences that impact on the reasoning process. Expertise in clinical reasoning relies on students being exposed to elements of both frames of reasoning processes.

USING THEORIES TO DRIVE EDUCATION METHODS

Example: When teaching and assessing a student's clinical reasoning skills, educators should provide them with opportunities to demonstrate an understanding of how the discrete elements of a patient's problem might lead to a particular clinical diagnosis. In addition, educators need to encourage students to think about and articulate how the broader social environment might influence their clinical decisions and clinical problem solving.

Introduction

In this chapter we examine current ideas about clinical reasoning, especially ideas such as what clinical reasoning is, and how it might be best learned and taught. This then informs the ways in which clinical reasoning may be developed in the clinical environment. Clinical reasoning is essentially concerned with the ways in which health practitioners think through the various clinical problems that confront them in their daily practice. However there are now a number of disparate ways of conceptualising clinical reasoning with widely differing assumptions of what is involved and what factors impact the process. This chapter focuses on two quite different, but related, approaches to clinical reasoning. The first approach is based on cognitive psychology and the second is from sociocultural studies.

Clinical reasoning has been the subject of research for several decades. How it is both conceptualised and researched has reflected the dominant paradigms of the times in which the research was done. The earliest research was conducted within the paradigm of behaviourism, followed soon after by its successor, cognitive science (Elstein et al 1990). In behaviourism and cognitivism there is an analytical focus on the changes occurring within the health professionals who are learning and doing the clinical reasoning. The focus is on the clinician as individual decision maker. The teaching of clinical reasoning within this paradigm naturally follows the imperative to bring about the required cognitive changes in newcomers to the health professions, who will then be able to behave appropriately (e.g. Custers & Boshuizen 2002).

In more recent years, different forms of research have emerged which stem from different sets of assumptions. These newer forms of research are based on more humanistic thinking from the humanities and social sciences. They have included research based on narrative thinking (Charon 2006, Mattingly 1994), professional artistry (Fish 1998), critical theory (Trede & Higgs 2003) and the use of language (Ajjawi 2006, Loftus 2006). These humanistic approaches can be included within the paradigm of interpretivism. Here, the analytical focus is much more on the social world within which clinical reasoning occurs, and the role of the clinician within this social world. In this chapter we synthesise current thinking about clinical reasoning within these different paradigms and present practical implications for developing clinical reasoning during clinical education. In order to do this, in the first half of the chapter the authors draw on models of reasoning founded in behaviourism and cognitivism and highlight the key features of 'the stage theory of expertise development' and acquisition in the health professions. The second half of the chapter focuses upon the interpretivist paradigm in clinical reasoning, and the strength of using narrative and sociological theory as a lens to view and better understand clinical reasoning in the healthcare setting.

Clinical reasoning as a cognitive phenomenon

There are many anecdotes about remarkable diagnosticians; physicians who do not heavily rely on inquiry because they already seem to 'know'. Can you imagine a scenario where the doctor is an elderly man who has been in family practice for about thirty years. He usually does not enquire very deeply into the nature of our symptoms; he appears absentminded when we present our complaints. He does not make an extensive use of diagnostic tools like laboratory tests or X-rays. And yet, he hardly ever misses a diagnosis. When we visit him with a penetrating pain in the chest, he does not refer us to the cardiologist but, after some questions, sends us home with the advice to take some rest because 'stress can do these things you know, but no doubt it will disappear in a few days'. And his advice turns out to be correct. When he sees our young daughter late in the evening having convulsions and a high fever, he decides to send her to the hospital but reassures us by saying that it does not seem to be something related to brain dysfunction, but rather the result of some infectious process, probably of urogenital origin. And his diagnosis proves to be accurate.

In this section of the chapter, we will discuss some of the reasons why experienced physicians display such remarkable diagnostic performance and how these skills have come to develop over the years in practice. The initial attempts to address these questions in the early 1970s, looked for expert doctors' superior reasoning *processes*. The well-known studies conducted by Elstein et al (1978) exemplify these 'processing theories'. They proposed the notion of the 'hypothetico-deductive method': early in the clinical encounter expert doctors generate diagnostic hypotheses and subsequently gather information to confirm or refute these hypotheses. Although this may describe the essential elements of the clinical reasoning process, it does not account for expert performance for a simple reason: subjects at all levels of expertise were shown to reason through similar processes.

As the idea of a general problem-solving process failed, research shifted towards 'structure theories', which focus on *underlying knowledge structures* that generate diagnostic hypotheses (Norman 2005, Ericsson 2007). Empirical research within this paradigm has concentrated on how expertise develops in medicine, by exploring how knowledge is acquired, organised in memory and used by experienced doctors for diagnosing clinical problems (Schmidt & Rikers 2007). These researchers generated a theory that considers the development of expertise as progressing through a number of transitory stages, each characterised by qualitatively different knowledge structures underlying diagnostic performance (Schmidt & Boshuizen 1993a, Schmidt et al 1990). In the next section, we sketch this theory and subsequently summarise findings of more recent studies that have clarified the process of clinicians' diagnostic reasoning. In the final section, we briefly discuss their implications for clinical education.

A stage theory of expertise development

Early theories of expertise development considered that students would turn into experts through extending their knowledge about relevant concepts in a domain and constructing meaningful relationships between them. Expertise would come, therefore, from *knowledge expansion*. In contrast, the stage theory presented here postulates that the development of expertise in medicine entails a process of *knowledge restructuring* in which students progress through four different stages in their growth towards expertise.

STAGE 1
In the course of the first years of their training, students rapidly develop rich, elaborated causal networks explaining the causes and consequences of diseases in terms of general underlying biological or pathophysiological processes.

The development of these causal networks can be illustrated by findings from a study by Schmidt et al (1988) in which students at different levels of training—first year health sciences students and second and fourth year medical students—were shown the case description in Box 7.1.

> **BOX 7.1** Case description of an acute endocarditis case
>
> A 27-year-old unemployed male was admitted to the emergency room. He complained of shaking chills and fever of four days' duration. He took his own temperature: it was recorded at 40°C on the morning of his admission. The fever and chills were accompanied by sweating, and a feeling of prostration. He also complained of some shortness of breath when he tried to climb the two flights of stairs in his apartment. The patient volunteered that he had been bitten by a cat at a friend's house a week before admission.
>
> Functional inquiry revealed a transient loss of vision in his right eye, which lasted approximately 45 seconds. This he described to have occurred in the day before admission to the emergence ward.
>
> Physical examination revealed a toxic looking young man who was having a rigor. His temperature was 41°C. Pulse was 124 per minute. BP 110/40. Mucous membranes were clear. Examination of his limbs showed puncture wounds in his left antecubital fossa. There were no other skin findings.
>
> Examination showed no jugular venous distention. Pulse was regular, equal and synchronous. The apex beat was not displaced. Auscultation of his heart revealed a 2/6 early diastolic murmur in the aortic area. Funduscopy revealed a flame-shaped haemorrhage in the left eye. There was no splenomegaly. Urinalysis showed numerous red cells. There were no red cell casts on microscopic urinalysis.

The students were asked to explain the signs and symptoms presented in the case (which is one of acute bacterial endocarditis due to intravenous drug use) in terms of the underlying pathophysiological processes. Analysis of the protocols generated by the three groups of students showed an almost linear increase in the number of propositions used to interpret the case.[1] This demonstrates the rapid development of elaborated causal networks explaining the causes and consequences of disease in terms of underlying pathophysiological processes.

Students at this stage of their education try to make sense of clinical cases presented to them by analysing isolated signs and symptoms and relating each of them with the pathophysiological mechanisms they have learned. As students do not yet recognise patterns of symptoms that fit together, processing of case information is effortful and detailed. This explains the 'intermediate effect' consistently found in the studies of clinical case recall, where intermediate-level students remember more details of cases than medical experts (Rikers et al 2000, Schmidt & Boshuizen 1993b). When asked to think aloud while solving cases, intermediate-level students were also shown to use detailed knowledge of the basic sciences in explaining for themselves the signs and symptoms of the patient. In contrast, references to basic science concepts were almost absent in think-aloud protocols of experienced doctors (Boshuizen & Schmidt 1992). This was thought to occur because the experienced doctors operate upon different

....

1 A proposition corresponds to a meaningful idea unit in the text and consists of two concepts linked by a qualifier, such as causation, specification, temporal information, or location (Patel & Groen 1986). For example, the fragment 'Pulse was regular' contains one proposition consisting of two concepts—pulse and regular—linked by a specification.

knowledge structures. This difference leads to the second stage in our theory of expertise development.

STAGE 2

Through extensive, repeated application of acquired knowledge and, particularly, exposure to patient problems, these elaborate networks of concepts and their interrelations become compiled into high-level, simplified causal models explaining signs and symptoms, and are subsumed under diagnostic labels (Boshuizen & Schmidt 1992).

The transition from the first to the second stage in students' knowledge structures (referred to as *knowledge encapsulation*) can be explained using data from the same study by Schmidt et al (1988). Box 7.2 displays the protocols produced by two medical students when they explained the case of endocarditis.

BOX 7.2 **Pathophysiology protocols of medical students at different levels of training**

PATHOPHYSIOLOGICAL PROTOCOL OF A FOURTH YEAR MEDICAL STUDENT
Probably this young man is an intravenous drug addict. And he is bitten by a cat. His resistance is not too good, so probably his immune system has not been able to eliminate the bacteria that have entered the man's body through the cat bite. As a consequence, his blood is invaded with bacteria. These bacteria produce toxins that are rendered harmless by antibodies. The complement system is activated and through this mechanism vasoactive substances are released, such as histamine and serotonin, etc. This is what is called the 'hot phase' of the septic shock. The temperature control centre is disturbed as well and is reset at a higher point. The body looses much heat and slowly the 'cold phase' of the anaphylactic shock is entered. This is characterised by shivers, pallor and a coldness of the extremities of the body, disseminated intravascular coagulation (because of a vicious circle in which several influences play a role, such as deteriorated oxygen supply, toxins, endothelium damage caused by a hypoxemia etc.). I think, ablatio retinae can be caused by this as well. At the moment of entrance his blood pressure was low (namely 110/40 mm Hg), then he was in the hot phase, in which reduced filling of the vascular bed caused this hypotension. Probably, the red cells in his urine can be explained by the disseminated intravascular coagulation that, accompanied with too much use of thrombocytes, causes a haemorrhagic diathesis; so this is caused by the consumption of platelets. In the end all organs are affected.

PATHOPHYSIOLOGICAL PROTOCOL OF AN INTERNIST
Through port of entry either venous punction or cat bite, a sepsis that secondary produces damages to the aortic valve (endocarditis), kidneys (glomerulonephritis), and the retina (extravasation of the blood in the retina).

The effects of compilation become evident when the two protocols are compared. The fourth year student used many words to explain the mechanisms involved in shock due to sepsis (in some respects, inadequately). The sixth year student did not refer to the word shock at all. The whole case was explained in terms of *sepsis* and its secondary effects. An internist would probably be even more concise and say: 'This drug user has developed a *sepsis* due to the use of contaminated needles'. Used in this way, the concept of *sepsis* encapsulates the fourth year student's detailed pathophysiological explanation. It is sufficient to fully explain the condition of the patient. Having a concept such as sepsis available to the reasoner enables them to see patterns of symptoms as wholes, considerably speeding up processing of a case, and adding to accurate diagnosis.

Several studies have confirmed the predictions derived from the notion that biomedical knowledge becomes encapsulated into clinical concepts. Pathophysiological explanations of experts were shown to contain less biomedical and more encapsulated concepts than those of students (Van de Wiel et al 2000), and recall protocols of experts contained more encapsulations than protocols of sub-experts (Rikers et al 2002). Experts have many encapsulating concepts available, describing syndromes or simplified causal mechanisms. This knowledge, often called *clinical knowledge* (as opposed to *biomedical knowledge*), tends to be used preferentially by experts (Boshuizen & Schmidt 1992, McLaughlin 2007). Indeed, biomedical knowledge apparently only indirectly relates to clinical competence (De Bruin et al 2005). Recent studies, however, have suggested that biomedical knowledge may play a more important role than is presently assumed (Woods et al 2005, 2006), but this requires further investigation.

Knowledge encapsulation, however, is not the last stage in the course towards expertise. A second transition in knowledge structures takes place when students enter into the clinical years.

STAGE 3

As students begin to practise extensively with patients, a second transition occurs, and their encapsulated knowledge reorganises into narrative structures called *illness scripts*. With growing experience with patients, the different ways by which disease manifests itself in varying signs and symptoms merge with pathophysiological knowledge, and students begin to pay attention to the contextual factors under which disease emerges. Instead of causal processes, the features that characterise the clinical appearance of a disease become the anchor points of their thinking. Gradually *illness scripts* for different diseases develop.

Illness scripts are cognitive structures containing relatively little knowledge about pathophysiological mechanisms, but a wealth of clinically relevant information about the disease (Feltovich & Barrows 1984). A general structure of an illness script consists of enabling conditions, faults and consequences. Enabling conditions are factors that generally make the occurrence of a certain disease or family of diseases more likely. The fault is a description of the malfunction, which may consist of a diagnostic label or a simplified description of a pathophysiological mechanism, for example, invasion of pathogenic organism into body tissue. The consequences generally are the signs and symptoms that arise from the fault (Feltovich & Barrows 1984).

Expertise development is associated with the emergence of illness scripts rich in knowledge of enabling conditions. Studies comparing students and physicians at different levels of expertise have shown that the number and richness of enabling conditions associated with particular diseases increase with expertise (Custers et al 1998), and experienced doctors tend to make extensive use of enabling conditions (Hobus 1994, Van Schaik et al 2005).

When physicians review a patient like the young man described in Box 7.1, they would search for an appropriate illness script in memory and when one (or a few) are selected, verify the script by matching its elements to the information provided by the patient. In this course of script verification, the script is said to become *instantiated*

(Schmidt & Rikers 2007, Schmidt & Boshuizen 1993b). These instantiated scripts do not necessarily become decontextualised but remain available in memory as episodic traces of previous patients. Illness scripts exist, therefore, at various levels of generality, ranging from representations of disease categories to prototypes, to representations of individual patients previously seen. Storing these different representations constitutes another transition, a fourth stage in the course of expertise development.

STAGE 4

Instantiated scripts generated during encounters with individual patients remain available in memory and may be used in the diagnosis of future similar problems. Experienced doctors' reasoning in routine situations is largely instance based.

Throughout years of clinical practice, doctors store in memory more and more instances of individual patients. Expert clinicians' reasoning is largely based on recognition of similarities between the case at hand and these examples of previous patients (Schmidt & Boshuizen 1993b, Schmidt et al 1990). This so-called *pattern-recognition reasoning* occurs in routine situations, rapidly and effortlessly, as a largely unconscious process without requiring physicians to analyse individual signs and symptoms or explain their causal mechanisms (Norman 2005, Norman & Brooks 1997, Ericsson 2004). Nevertheless, the knowledge structures acquired in the earlier stages of expertise development, such as pathophysiological knowledge, do not decay but remain available in memory and may be activated when pattern-recognition reasoning fails (Schmidt & Boshuizen 1993a, Schmidt et al 1990, Patel & Groen 1986).

The role of experience and examples of prior patients in diagnostic reasoning

The influence of prior examples on the generation of diagnostic hypotheses was first demonstrated by empirical studies in the domain of dermatology conducted by Brooks, Norman and colleagues in the 1980s (Brooks et al 1991). Medical students were asked to diagnose dermatological conditions, and similarity with a previously seen example of the particular condition was shown to dramatically influence diagnostic accuracy. Subsequent studies in other domains, such as electrocardiography and psychiatry, reaffirmed non-analytical reasoning based on similarity to prior examples as a crucial component of diagnostic reasoning (Hatala et al 1999, Norman et al 2007). Moreover studies have shown that, far from being objective, interpretation of signs and symptoms in a case tends to be influenced by the diagnosis under consideration. When medical students were presented with photographs of classical signs of diseases, features were shown to be easily misinterpreted due to the influence of an initial hypothesis (LeBlanc et al 2002).

These findings raise the question of how reasoning strategies affect the quality of diagnoses. Studies on diagnostic errors have pointed to the negative consequences of relying excessively on non-analytical reasoning (Croskerry 2003, Graber et al 2002). Diagnostic errors derived from premature closure, which seem to increase with ageing, exemplify these possible deleterious effects (Eva 2002). Apparently non-analytical reasoning is highly effective in routine situations but may provoke failures when doctors encounter complex or unusual problems (Ericsson 2004, Croskerry 2005). Concerns with avoidable medical errors have contributed to attention being directed to the other pole of the spectrum of diagnostic reasoning. It is known that expert doctors may shift from the usual automatic way of reasoning to an analytical, effortful diagnostic approach in some situations (Patel & Groen 1986, Rikers et al 2002). This has been reported when doctors diagnose cases outside of their own domain of expertise; in such cases they adopted an elaborate biomedical processing approach for understanding signs and symptoms (Rikers et al 2002).

Some of our recent empirical studies have confirmed that doctors may engage in effortful reflection for diagnosing cases (Mamede & Schmidt 2004, Mamede et al 2007). Findings of these studies shed light on the analytical mode of diagnostic reasoning and will be briefly discussed here.

The nature of reflective reasoning and its effect on diagnoses

Reflective practice can be conceptualised as the ability of health practitioners to critically reflect on their own reasoning and decisions (Mamede & Schmidt 2004), and has a multidimensional structure. It implies an openness to recognising difficulties, thereby engaging in reflection, and it involves an elaborate, careful consideration of case findings, while critically scrutinising one's own reasoning (Mamede & Schmidt 2004).

Recent empirical studies with internal medicine residents have explored the effects of the two main modes of reasoning on quality of diagnoses. Residents were asked to diagnose simple and complex cases by following instructions that led either to a non-analytical or a reflective approach. Reflection improved accuracy of diagnoses in complex cases whereas it made no difference in diagnoses of simple cases (Mamede et al 2008). A second study with medical residents reaffirmed this positive effect of reflective reasoning on the diagnosis of difficult, ambiguous clinical cases (Mamede et al, in press). The implication of these findings is that diagnostic decisions could be improved by adjusting reasoning approaches to situational demands. This finding also raises the question of how experienced physicians, who tend to reason highly automatically, recognise when a problem requires further reflection. Studies have shown that physicians in fact shift to analytical approaches (Mamede & Schmidt 2004, Rikers et al 2002), but conditions under which this occurs are still under investigation. Complexity of the case to be diagnosed seems to be one of these conditions (Mamede et al 2007). Contextual information may also trigger reflection. In another study with residents, knowledge that other physicians had previously incorrectly diagnosed the case led participants to adopt a reflective approach (Mamede et al, in press).

Over the past decades a variety of studies have contributed to clarify the kinds of knowledge used in non-analytical reasoning. We know very little, however, about the knowledge structures and mental processes involved when physicians process clinical cases in a reflective mode. In our studies, when medical residents engaged in reflection for diagnosing cases they used findings presented in case description, that is patient medical history or contextual information, signs, and symptoms, more extensively and made more inferences about pathophysiological mechanisms and alternative diagnoses (Mamede et al, in press). However the role of each kind of knowledge in generation and verification of diagnostic hypotheses, and how they affect diagnostic accuracy, requires further investigation.

Research on clinical reasoning started with attempts to reveal general problem-solving strategies used by experts with the aim of teaching them to students. When it became clear that no superior reasoning processes characterised expertise, attention was reoriented to types of knowledge and mental representations. With the recent studies on reflective reasoning, it may seem that we have turned back to the starting point by focusing again on reasoning strategies. These are not, however, general, knowledge-independent strategies, but instead strategies to access and use the different knowledge structures available in physicians' memory relevant to a particular patient or illness script. Students' or physicians' ability to use a certain reasoning strategy does not develop, therefore, in isolation, but depends on the acquisition of the knowledge to be applied with this strategy.

Implications for clinical education

Research on cognitive processes in clinical reasoning has generated a substantial amount of empirical evidence about how practitioners make diagnoses. What emerges from these studies as recommendations that may improve clinical education include, first, that teaching basic and clinical sciences should be integrated around organ systems or problems. Second, to provide support to the development of encapsulating concepts, curricula should facilitate the formation of illness scripts. Students should have the opportunity to work with patient problems early in the curriculum, and should encounter many patients. Not only patients with a diversity of problems, but many examples of how the same disease may present itself in daily life.

Third, feedback and support for reflection are likely to facilitate the process of knowledge encapsulation, formation of illness scripts, and storing of instantiated scripts. In clinical settings students should have time to elaborate on the problems of the patients they encounter, and support for reflection. By reflecting on a patient with a preceptor or in small groups of peers, students could better apprehend, for instance, enabling conditions encountered in that particular patient or a variant of a disease presentation. Further research is required to explore whether and how strategies aimed at promoting reflection in clinical teaching (Smith & Irby 1997, Ferenchick et al 1997) could be used to facilitate the development of knowledge structures and reasoning processes in novice practitioners.

Clinical reasoning as an interpretive phenomenon

A growing dissatisfaction with the cognitive-behavioural paradigm described above has encouraged many researchers in recent years to adopt approaches from the social sciences and humanities when thinking about clinical reasoning (Higgs et al 2008). The dissatisfaction is due to a number of reasons. For example, much of the research in clinical reasoning has focused on clinico-pathological diagnosis. For health workers in fields like occupational therapy such research is largely irrelevant. The work of occupational therapists begins after a clinico-pathological diagnosis has been made. Occupational therapists focus on rehabilitation. This is why a narrative approach was used by Mattingly (1994) to look into how occupational therapists thought through clinical problems. The idea of narrative in clinical reasoning is being rapidly adopted throughout the health professions as it provides a conceptually rich way of thinking about what constitutes clinical reasoning.

There are many similarities between the notions of illness scripts and narrative. Greenhalgh (1999) discusses an experienced doctor very similar to the one described above. However, Greenhalgh describes the doctor's expertise in terms of deep narrative knowing. It can be argued that the notion of narrative subsumes that of an illness script. The major difference is that an illness script is seen as being something exclusively inside a clinician's head, whereas narrative goes beyond this and explores how the patient's story can be jointly constructed by the patient and health professional. This is especially important in rehabilitation where patients or clients must work together with health professionals if there is to be a successful outcome. However it is now realised that a narrative approach can be applied to all healthcare settings.

Narrative medicine

Mattingly (1994) introduced the notion of 'therapeutic emplotment', providing a detailed example of how this was seen in the clinical setting. She described an occupational therapist taking a new patient for a tour around a rehabilitation facility, showing him where various activities would take place. It is clear from Mattingly's analysis that the therapist's talk was attempting to lay down a new narrative foundation for the patient. A young, previously able-bodied person now had to learn to live the rest of his life in a disabled state. This meant working out and living a new narrative, and the therapist clearly attempted to provide the beginnings of a narrative in which the patient had a meaningful life and coped with his disabilities. In other words, the therapist provided the plot that the new narrative might follow—if the patient accepted it. Mattingly argued that without this larger therapeutic story the clinical encounters of rehabilitation would become meaningless, and patients (and presumably staff) would see little purpose in engaging in therapy at all.

Loftus (2006) made similar findings in his study of a pain clinic where it was clear that the rehabilitation program encouraged patients to live out a new narrative where chronic pain was an accepted part of life, but managed, and kept in the background. Even though the pain clinic used the discourse of cognitive behavioural therapy, it was clear that the activity of the clinic could be richly described in narrative terms. Patients suffering from chronic pain were living out narratives of steady deterioration in which jobs were lost and relationships ruined. The therapy of the pain clinic encouraged patients to collaborate with the health professionals to work out new meaningful stories, customised for each individual. For example, if a patient's ambition was to return to a particular job then a therapeutic program was devised that worked towards this specific goal, in addition to providing general coping strategies. It was a goal that meant the therapy became meaningful to the patient, a part of their new life story. However narrative is relevant in both acute and chronic settings.

Advocates of a narrative approach (Charon 2006, Greenhalgh 1998, Greenhalgh et al 2004) argue that a large part of medicine (and all healthcare) is narrative construction. Making a diagnosis is reinterpreting patients' stories within the terminology of medicine. For example, a patient who presents with a story of acute toothache may be assessed and given a diagnosis of impacted wisdom teeth. The story of impacted wisdom teeth is the same narrative reinterpreted in medical terms. The strength of the reinterpreted medical narrative is that it suggests a narrative trajectory into the future. In this example, surgical removal of the wisdom teeth would result in a satisfactory ending to the story. Diseases and disorders can be thought of as following narrative forms, and thinking of clinico-pathological conditions in terms of the story-lines they tend to follow can be a powerful way of learning about healthcare.

It is important to realise that allowing patients to tell their stories can be powerfully therapeutic. Charon (2006) relates how she gives patients time to tell their stories in their own words, without interruption, and the positive ways in which patients react to this. Frank (1995, 2005) also spoke of the need for patients, especially those with chronic conditions, to be given the chance to tell their stories and be believed. Loftus (2006) found many patients in the pain clinic he studied felt 'validated' by the opportunity they were given to tell their stories in full. They needed what Kleinman (1988) called empathic witnessing, the need to be heard and understood.

Greenhalgh (1999) described the diagnostic encounter as being an occasion in which a number of separate secondary texts are integrated into one narrative. She described these secondary texts as:

- the experiential text—the meaning patients assign to their problems
- the narrative text—the medical history and its interpretation by the doctor
- the physical text—what the physical examination reveals
- the instrumental text—information from special tests like radiographs.

Greenhalgh contended that special tests like radiographs, biopsies and blood tests can rarely be interpreted in isolation. They need an accompanying medical and social history if they are to be interpreted adequately. This is consistent with Montgomery's (2006) notion of medicine as a hermeneutic (interpretive) practice. Each text is a part that needs to be integrated into a narrative whole.

Greenhalgh (1999) discussed the ways in which narrative medicine could be combined with modern scientific trends, such as the evidence-based medicine (EBM) movement. She saw them not as necessarily contradictory but as complementary. EBM is used to study populations, but narratives refer to individual cases. Greenhalgh made the sensible proposition that both kinds of knowledge are needed in modern medical practice.

Narrative is just one example of the ways in which ideas from the humanities and social sciences have started to change the ways in which we think about clinical reasoning. For a fuller picture of how the social sciences can inform clinical reasoning see Higgs et al (2008). Looking at clinical reasoning from the interpretive paradigm is relatively new, and there is limited research from this perspective when compared to the cognitivist perspective. However, the interpretive paradigm is opening up a vast new research agenda for investigating clinical reasoning in all the health professions. The kind of research opened up by a narrative approach to clinical reasoning includes questions such as: In what ways does a narrative approach change how clinicians view the process of diagnosis and prognosis? And in what ways is patient care changed by clinicians adopting a narrative approach to clinical reasoning? Next we look at how the teaching of clinical reasoning can be approached using a humanistic social science framework.

Clinical education for clinical reasoning

Despite the differences in how clinical reasoning is conceptualised, there appears to be a great deal of convergence between the two approaches when it comes to how clinical reasoning can and should be taught. Proponents of both approaches now advocate educational methods that put students in real, or realistic, scenarios reflecting real-world practice as much as possible. Therefore approaches, such as problem- or case-based learning and clinical attachments, where students can participate in the practice of clinical reasoning, are seen as being ideal educational situations. It is important for students to actively participate rather than merely observe whenever possible. The rest of this chapter expands upon one particular way of conceptualising learning of clinical reasoning in which students are gradually socialised into the communities of practice called healthcare professions.

Learning to reason as a journey of professional socialisation: a reconceptualisation

Professional socialisation is an ideal framework for conceptualising how health professionals learn to reason in the clinical setting (Ajjawi & Higgs 2008). Key research findings to support this view are that experienced physiotherapists develop their reasoning capability in context supported by their professional communities of practice (Ajjawi 2006). Clinical reasoning is embedded in the context of professional practice and is, therefore, best learned in the very same context where individuals are developing and becoming members of the profession. Clinical education provides novice health professionals with opportunities to practise reasoning and its communication with a wide variety of patients. This is a potent aid to their development of clinical reasoning ability.

The term journey is used here to highlight the fact that professional socialisation is not a single event (Richardson 1999a, b) but rather the ongoing development of individuals through repeated interactions with their environment. Clinical reasoning is a prime example of an ability that emerges in this way (Ajjawi & Higgs 2008). Students enter as adult learners with general problem-solving skills; they then learn how the profession reasons and deals with the tasks and challenges of professional practice. Clinical reasoning ability continues to develop following graduation through ongoing formal and informal education, reflection on experience, self-directed learning and learning from others (such as through the mentoring process or from supportive peers) (Ajjawi 2006). Aspects of this journey may be both implicit and explicit.

Professional socialisation is not simply a passive process of internalisation. There is individual agency for what one takes on board and what is disregarded (Clouder 2003). Judgements about the suitability or appropriateness of what is modelled by others is processed against the individual's frame of reference, values, beliefs, and sense of self as a person and as a professional (McArdle & Coutis 2003). In these judgements, clinicians apply professional, critical and ethical judgements to construct new meanings in response to new challenges and situations. Although learning to reason may often be subconscious (Ajjawi & Higgs 2008), it is not passive. Modelling of behaviour requires active interpretation and integration of the processes perceived as useful or relevant by the learner (Bandura 1971). In her research, Ajjawi found that learning to reason required a mixture of enhanced awareness and monitoring, deliberate paying attention and collaborative learning relationships within supportive practice communities.

Learning in communities of practice and the emphasis on the cultural learning process can be seen as essential parts of the broader concept of professional socialisation (Abrandt Dahlgren et al 2004). Clinical education is the natural setting for such communities which include patients, caregivers, colleagues and other health professionals. Learning is enhanced through participation in everyday work practices where the contexts of learning and practice are identical. Formation of a professional identity with professional responsibilities, including accountability and duty of care for patients, motivates such learning. Health professionals are further motivated to improve their reasoning and communication abilities when facing challenging work situations that stretch them in their 'zones of proximal development' (Vygotsky 1978), that is, when the situation offers challenges that are beyond what they can accomplish independently. This is when peers, role models and mentors function to extend or scaffold learning through guidance, modelling, discussion and feedback in the context of the challenging situation.

Learning within communities of practice is a move away from the apprenticeship model as students are no longer solely dependent on one clinical educator for their learning. Developing learning communities within healthcare teams distributes the responsibility for mentoring and support across multiple health professionals. Such communities function with teaching and learning as primary goals for everyone, embedded in daily practice rather than being additional responsibilities or chores. Learning occurs through legitimate participation in the daily activities of the community (Lave & Wenger 1991). Involving students in team clinical reasoning, for example, can be a powerful learning experience. However this might require a different model for student assessment than current practice, one that accounts for feedback from the different members involved in student learning with an emphasis on capturing the range of interpersonal interactions in context (Kuper et al 2007).

Implications for the role of clinical educators

The implications for adopting a sociocultural rather than a purely cognitive perspective on clinical reasoning are a strong emphasis on the role of clinical education in the socialisation of future health professionals. Clinical education provides an environment in which learners can engage in purposeful activities with real and realistic goals. In the process, they learn to use the cultural tools and practices that have been developed to meet those goals. The jargon used by health professionals in reasoning and communicating reasoning is an example of a culturally mediated tool (Loftus 2006) that can and should be learned in the clinical environment. Learning the language of clinical reasoning serves to shape our thoughts and ideas; teaching novices how to talk about their practice helps them learn how to think about their patients and their work (Lingard & Haber 1999). By telling stories and learning the language, novices construct identities as members of that community (Brown & Duguid 1991), allowing them to gain entry and participate in the practices of the community (Lave & Wenger 1991), which begins the acculturation process.

Clinical educators need to be aware of their professional responsibilities in guiding and mentoring the development of clinical reasoning in novice practitioners, and provide a dynamic, responsible and supportive learning community. It is important to acknowledge that the knowledge, skills and, in particular, the attitudes of senior colleagues or role models strongly influence the development of students' professional identities (Higgs 1993). This influence transcends what is articulated explicitly; it includes the behaviour and values that embody a profession, which may be implicit or tacit, but remain highly influential in learning and professional development.

In generating effective learning communities, clinical educators can make novices feel that it is appropriate to ask questions about why certain things are done in the everyday work environment (Hoff et al 2004). They should also consider the impact on novices if they are not accepted into the community of practice, of being marginalised, and the significant impact on the development of a professional identity and the socialisation process. Coulehan (2005) called for practitioners to model professional virtue at every stage of health professional education in order to engender professionalism in novice practitioners. Such virtues encompass integrity in interactions with patients, staff, colleagues and the community, and a broad humanistic and narrative perspective. Coulehan also urged experienced practitioners to provide safe environments for novice practitioners to share their experiences and enhance their awareness of their practice.

The role of the clinical educator in developing novice reasoning includes finding the 'optimum' balance between challenge and support. Actively reasoning about challenging cases, considering alternative courses of action, and applying and evaluating the reasoned solution focuses attention onto the process of clinical reasoning (Ajjawi & Higgs 2008). During clinical education, novices can be helped to recognise when situations are outside their ability to solve, which should then lead to self-directed learning through review of journal articles or seeking help from more capable or expert persons. All professionals need to strive for continuous monitoring and awareness in their practice of clinical reasoning, in order to address emergent difficulties and limitations (Eva & Regehr 2005). In this way, reflexivity and lifelong, self-directed learning skills foster the development of reasoning skills. Reflexivity is evident in heightened awareness and self-critique of practice, with a genuine desire to continue to improve. It is evident in a constant questioning stance or a state of 'mindfulness' (Epstein 1999), and is arguably an important ability to develop through interaction with reflexive therapists and socialisation during clinical education.

Another role for clinical educators is to focus novice practitioners' attention towards salient cognitive and contextual features of a current activity. Feedback on clinical reasoning is necessary to inform learners' ability to judge their actions and decisions relative to a particular situation. This is particularly relevant as self-assessment does not appear to be a stable, global skill that is easily acquired or developed, but rather is situationally bound and context specific (Eva & Regehr 2005). Therefore, strategies that can be used to facilitate novices learning of reasoning include modelling, guiding, discussion, articulating reasoning paths and the values and beliefs informing judgements and decisions, providing feedback and guiding reflection. These strategies are congruent with learning in communities of practice because of the emphasis on collaborative learning through social participation, dialogue and negotiation.

It can be argued from much clinical reasoning research that there is no one generic reasoning strategy. This is not just because reasoning is based on an individual's knowledge base, but also because of the unique interpretation of reasoning by each therapist for each patient and each situation. Various authors have documented aspects of these essential qualities of reasoning (e.g. Eva 2004, Higgs & Jones 2008). Therefore clinical educators need to articulate their reasoning clearly when communicating reasoning with novice physiotherapists, who may assume invalid links between knowledge and data if only the decision (or product of reasoning) is articulated. Learning and teaching of clinical reasoning should focus on facilitating and developing unique reasoning ability in others, rather than expecting them to adopt a direct teaching or knowledge transfer approach. It is important to help novice practitioners develop strategies to deal with the varied demands that different situations place on reasoning task. The following points provide a summary list of key methods to promote, facilitate and develop reasoning abilities through clinical education:

- facilitating the development of clinical reasoning should be an explicit aim of clinical education
- clinical educators play an active role in the acculturation of students: this encompasses modelling of the values, beliefs and attitudes of the profession
- participation in legitimate decision-making activities of the community is ideal for novice reasoners to learn to reason
- strategies that promote the development of reasoning include guidance, discussion of thinking and decision-making processes, reflection and feedback
- encouraging articulation of thinking processes increases awareness of own clinical reasoning
- students can be guided to become aware of influence of contextual factors in the clinical reasoning process
- clinical reasoning requires interpretive and narrative capabilities as well as cognitive capabilities—students need to be guided in developing social, interactive and emotional capabilities.

The value and complexity of communicating clinical reasoning

Reconceptualising the development of clinical reasoning within the framework of professional socialisation highlights the importance of learning to communicate reasoning during clinical education. The implication is that learning to reason is not only an individual process; it is also a social process. Learning from peers is a powerful way to learn to reason through discussion, both formal and informal. Health professionals learn to articulate, critique and defend their reasoning through conversations and reflection with peers, about real patient cases (Ajjawi 2006). The process of articulating reasoning draws clinical reasoning, a skill that is often subconscious, to the participants' awareness, making it explicit and thereby exposing it to self-critique, and critique and feedback from others. Articulating reasoning helps professionals learn to reason better.

This finding aligns with Vygotsky's (1978) notion that higher psychological functions (such as clinical reasoning) are developed by social interaction through the medium of language, both spoken and written (see further discussion in Ch 4). Therefore the process of learning to reason is mediated through discussions with peers and more expert colleagues about patient cases, using specific language such as professional 'jargon' that facilitates communication of these ideas. Language serves to shape our thoughts and ideas (Lingard & Haber 1999). According to Vygotsky (1986), language and consciousness are intimately woven within social activities and interactions. Situations in which people are required to articulate their thoughts and justify their opinions provide opportunities to analyse thought processes: language and thought are interdependent.

However articulating reasoning does not necessarily reflect actual reasoning processes because reasoning is rapid, situated and involves tacit knowledge. Communication of reasoning represents a reconstruction of the main processes perceived as most relevant to the audience, framed and delivered to match the audience (Ajjawi & Higgs 2008). Students need to learn to become aware of their thinking and to be given the necessary tools to construct their messages, including active listening, skills in interpersonal communication and collaborating with others. In addition, learning environments should provide safety in learning situations, allowing students to articulate inaccurate or 'messy' thinking without fear of embarrassment or negative consequences.

We are only now beginning to appreciate the extent to which linguistic and discursive forms, such as narrative, form a part of the phenomenon of clinical reasoning (Loftus 2006). This exciting research agenda can help us explore questions such as: What language tools need to be acquired and used when health professionals are required to make decisions in interprofessional contexts? And how does identity formation in novice health professionals influence the development of clinical reasoning (and vice versa)?

Conclusion

We have presented multiple models of clinical reasoning that work at different levels of abstraction. In this sense clinical reasoning is a little like biology. Biology can be studied at several levels of abstraction from ecosystems to molecular biology. It is inappropriate to ask which model is 'better' or closer to the truth. It all depends on the purpose for which the model is to be used. If our purpose is to undertake genetic engineering then a molecular biology model is appropriate. If our purpose is to manage water resources in a mountain range then an ecosystem model is appropriate. Clinical reasoning is similar. If our goal as clinical educators is to bring about cognitive change in our students, such as encouraging them to use the hypothetico-deductive approach, then a cognitive model will be appropriate. If our goal is to bring students into a community of professional practice, then a sociocultural approach is a more appropriate way of thinking through the issues we face. The settings in which we find ourselves as clinical educators may require that we use all the models at various times. Illness scripts and narrative may have something in common but emphasise quite different aspects of clinical reasoning.

Again, asking which is 'true' may be inappropriate. Asking which is more useful may be a more interesting question, and the answer may vary depending on the context. Clinical educators will need to find their own answers. The field of clinical reasoning is at an interesting stage. There is a rich variety of thinking about what it is and how it might best be taught. Clinical educators need to be aware of the different approaches and exercise their own judgement as to which model to use in any given situation.

References

Abrandt Dahlgren M, Richardson B, Sjostrom B 2004 Professions as communities of practice. In: Higgs J, Richardson B, Abrandt Dahlgren M (eds) Developing practice knowledge for health professionals. Butterworth-Heinemann, Edinburgh, p 71–88

Ajjawi R 2006 Learning to communicate clinical reasoning in physiotherapy practice. Faculty of Health Sciences, University of Sydney. Online. Available: http://hdl.handle.net/2123/1556 Accessed 9 Jan 2009

Ajjawi R, Higgs J 2008 Learning to reason: a journey of professional socialisation. Advances in Health Sciences Education Theory and Practice 13(2):133–150

Bandura A 1971 Analysis of modeling processes. In: Bandura A (ed) Psychological modelling. Aldine Atherton, Chicago, p 1–62

Boshuizen HPA, Schmidt HG 1992 On the role of biomedical knowledge in clinical reasoning by experts, intermediates and novices. Cognitive Science 16(2):153–184

Brooks LR, Norman GR, Allen SW 1991 The role of specific similarity in a medical diagnostic task. Journal of Experimental Psychology–Gen 120:278–287

Brown JS, Duguid P 1991 Organizational learning and communities-of-practice: toward a unified view of working, learning, and innovation. Organization Science 2(1):40–57

Charon R 2006 Narrative medicine: honoring the stories of illness. Oxford University Press, UK

Clouder L 2003 Becoming professional: exploring the complexities of professional socialisation in health and social care. Learning in Health and Social Care, 2(4):213–222

Coulehan J 2005 Today's professionalism: engaging the mind but not the heart. Academic Medicine 80(10):892–898

Croskerry P 2003 The importance of cognitive errors in diagnosis and strategies to minimise them. Academic Medicine 78:775–780

Croskerry P 2005 The theory and practice of clinical decision-making. Canadian Journal of Anesthiology 52(6):R1–R8

Custers E, Boshiuzen HPA 2002 The psychology of learning. In: Norman GR, van der Vleuten CPM, Newble DI (eds), International handbook of research in medical education. Kluwer Academic, Dordrecht/Boston/London, 1:163–204

Custers E, Boshiuzen HPA, Schmidt HG 1998 The role of illness scripts in the development of medical diagnostic expertise: results from an interview study. Cognition and instruction 16(4):367–398

De Bruin ABH, Schmidt HG, Rikers RMJP 2005 The role of basic science knowledge and clinical knowledge in diagnostic reasoning: a structural equation modeling approach. Academic Medicine 80(8):765–773

Elstein AS, Shulman LS, Sprafka SA 1978 Medical problem solving: an analysis of clinical reasoning. Harvard University Press, Cambridge, MA

Elstein AS, Shulman L, Sprafka SA 1990 Medical problem solving: a ten year retrospective. Evaluation and the Health Professions 13(1):5–36

Epstein RM 1999 Mindful practice. Journal of the American Medical Association 282(9): 833–839

Ericsson KA 2004 Deliberate practice and the acquisition and maintenance of expert performance in medicine and related domains. Academic Medicine 79(10):S70–81

Ericsson KA 2007 An expert-performance perspective of research on medical expertise: the study of clinical performance. Medical Education 41:1124–1130

Eva KW 2002 The aging physician: changes in cognitive processing and their impact on medical practice. Academic Medicine 77(10 Suppl):S1–6

Eva KW 2004 What every teacher needs to know about clinical reasoning. Medical Education 39(1):98–106

Eva KW, Regehr G 2005 Self-assessment in the health professions: a reformulation and research agenda. Academic Medicine 80(10 suppl):S46–54

Feltovich PJ, Barrows HS 1984 Issues of generality in medical problem solving. In: Schmidt HG, de Volder ML (eds) Tutorials in problem-based learning. Van Gorcum, Assen/Maastricht, Netherlands

Ferenchick G, Simpson D, Blackman J et al 1997 Strategies for efficient and effective teaching in the ambulatory care setting. Academic Medicine 72(4):277–280

Fish D 1998 Appreciating practice in the caring professions: re-focusing professional research and development. Elsevier, London

Frank AW 1995 The wounded storyteller: body, illness, and ethics. University of Chicago Press, Chicago

Frank A 2005 The renewal of generosity: illness, medicine and how to live. University of Chicago Press, Chicago

Graber M, Gordon R, Franklin N 2002 Reducing diagnostic errors in medicine: what's the goal? Academic Medicine 77:981–992

Greenhalgh T 1999 Narrative based medicine: narrative based medicine in an evidence based world. British Medical Journal 318:323–325

Greenhalgh T (ed) 1998 Narrative based medicine: dialogue and discourse in clinical practice. BMJ Books, London

Greenhalgh T, Hurwitz B, Skultans V (eds) 2004 Narrative research in health and illness. BMJ Books, London

Hatala RM, Norman GR, Brooks LR 1999 Influence of a single example upon subsequent electrocardiogram interpretation. Teaching and Learning in Medicine 11:110–117

Higgs J 1993 Physiotherapy, professionalism and self-directed learning. Journal of Singapore Physiotherapy Association 14(1):8–11

Higgs J, Jones M 2008 Clinical decision making and multiple problem spaces. In: Higgs J, Jones M, Loftus S et al (eds) Clinical reasoning in the health professions, 3rd edn. Butterworth-Heinemann, Oxford, p 3–18

Higgs J, Jones M, Loftus S et al (eds) 2008 Clinical reasoning in the health professions, 3rd edn. Butterworth-Heinemann, Oxford

Hobus PPM 1994 Expertise van huisartsen, praktijkervaring, kennis en diagnostische hypothesevorming (Expertise of family physicians; practical experience, knowledge and the formation of diagnostic hypotheses). University of Limburg, Maastrich, The Netherlands

Hoff TJ, Pohl H, Bartfield J 2004 Creating a learning environment to produce competent residents: the roles of culture and context. Academic Medicine 79(6):532–540

Kleineman A 1988 The illness narratives: Suffering, healing and the human condition. Basic Books, New York

Kuper A, Reeves S, Albert M et al 2007 Assessment: do we need to broaden our methodological horizons? Medical Education 41(12):1121–1123

Lave J, Wenger E 1991 Situated learning: legitimate peripheral participation. Cambridge University Press, UK

LeBlanc VR, Brooks LR, Norman GR 2002 Believing is seeing: the influence of a diagnostic hypothesis on the interpretation of clinical features. Academic Medicine 77(Suppl):67–69

Lingard L, Haber RJ 1999 Teaching and learning communication in medicine: a rhetorical approach. Academic Medicine 74(5):507–510

Loftus S 2006 Language in clinical reasoning: using and learning the language of collective clinical decision making. University of Sydney, Sydney. Online. Available: http://hdl.handle.net/2123/1165 9 Jan 2009

Mamede S, Schmidt HG 2004 The structure of reflective practice in medicine. Medical Education 38:1302–1308

Mamede S, Schmidt HG, Penaforte JC 2008 Effects of reflective practice on the accuracy of medical diagnoses. Medical Education 42(5):468–475

Mamede SM, Schmidt HG, Rikers RMJP et al 2007 Breaking down automaticity: case ambiguity and shift to reflective approaches in clinical reasoning. Medical Education 41:1185–1192

Mamede S, Schmidt HG, Rikers RMJP et al (in press) Influence of perceived difficulty of cases on physicians' diagnostic reasoning

Mattingly C 1994 The concept of therapeutic 'emplotment'. Social Science & Medicine 38:811–822

McArdle K, Coutis N 2003 A strong core of qualities: a model of the professional educator that moves beyond reflection. Studies in Continuing Education, 25(2):225–237

McLaughlin KJ 2007 The contribution of analytic information processing to diagnostic performance in medicine. Erasmus University, Rotterdam

Montgomery K 2006 How doctors think: clinical judgment and the practice of medicine. Oxford University Press, New York

Norman G 2005 Research in clinical reasoning: past history and current trends. Medical Education 39:418–427

Norman G, Young M, Brooks L 2007 Non-analytical models of clinical reasoning: the role of experience. Medical Education 41:1140–1145

Norman GR, Brooks LR 1997 The non-analytical basis of clinical reasoning. Advances in Health Science Education Theory and Practice 2:173–184

Patel VL, Groen GJ 1986 Knowledge-based solution strategies in medical reasoning. Cognitive Science 10:91–116

Richardson B 1999a Professional development: professional socialisation and professionalisation. Physiotherapy 85(9):461–467

Richardson B 1999b Professional development: professional knowledge and situated learning in the workplace. Physiotherapy 85(9):467–474

Rikers RMJP, Schmidt HG, Boshuizen HPA 2000 Knowledge encapsulation and the intermediate effect. Contemporary Educational Psychology 25(2):150–166

Rikers RMJP, Schmidt HG, Boshuizen HPA 2002 On the constraints of encapsulated knowledge: clinical case representations by medical experts and subexperts. Cognition and Instruction 20(1):27–45

Schmidt HG, Boshuizen HPA, Hobus PPM 1988 Transitory stages in the development of medical expertise: the 'intermediate effect' in clinical case representation studies. Proceedings of the Tenth Annual Conference of the Cognitive Science Society, Montreal, Canada. Erlbaum, Hillsdale, NJ

Schmidt HG, Boshuizen HPA 1993a On acquiring expertise in medicine. Educational Psychology Review 5:1–17

Schmidt HG, Boshuizen HPA 1993b On the origin of intermediate effects in clinical case recall. Memory & Cognition 21(3):338–351

Schmidt HG, Norman GR, Boshuizen HPA 1990 Cognitive Perspective on Medical Expertise: Theory and Implications. Academic Medicine 65(10):611–621

Schmidt HG, Rikers RMJP 2007 How expertise develops in medicine: knowledge encapsulation and illness script formation. Medical Education 41:1133–1139

Smith CS, Irby DM 1997 The roles of experience and reflection in ambulatory care education. Academic Medicine 72:32–35

Trede F, Higgs J 2003 Reframing the clinician's role in collaborative clinical decision making: rethinking practice knowledge and the notion of clinician–patient relationships. Learning in Health and Social Care 2:66–73

van de Wiel MWJ, Boshuizen HPA, Schmidt HG 2000 Knowledge restructuring in expertise development: evidence from pathophysiological representations of clinical cases by students and physicians. European Journal of Cognitive Psychology 12(3):323–355

van Schaik P, Flynn D, van Wersch A et al 2005 Influence of illness script components and medical practice on medical decision making. Journal of Experimental Psychology–Applied 11(3):187–199

Vygotsky LS 1978 Mind in society: the development of higher psychological processes. trans. M Cole. Harvard University Press, Cambridge

Vygotsky LS 1986 Thought and language. trans. A Kozulin. MIT Press, Cambridge

Woods NN, Brooks LR, Norman GR 2005 The value of basic science in clinical diagnosis: creating coherence among signs and symptoms. Medical Education 39(1):107–112

Woods NN, Neville AJ, Levinson AJ et al 2006 The value of basic science in clinical diagnosis. Academic Medicine 81(10):S124–S127

CHAPTER 8

Time to pause: giving and receiving feedback in clinical education

Elizabeth Molloy

THEORIES

In this chapter *Positioning Theory* (Harré & van Langenhove 1999) is applied as an analytical lens to study how students and educators interact in verbal feedback encounters. Positioning theory highlights the fine-grained social mechanics of the feedback sessions, and the mutually constructed and sanctioned 'roles' within the educational relationship. In addition, theories of critical reflection resonate through out the chapter, and underpin the practical recommendations for improving student agency, and feedback delivery and utility in clinical education.

USING THEORIES TO INFORM CURRICULUM DESIGN AND RESEARCH

Educators need to understand the positions they are adopting and projecting when giving feedback to students. It is also important to recognise the tendency for students to view the educator as 'diagnostician' and to adopt the counter position of 'passive recipient' during the sessions. The interactive and dialogic dimensions in feedback sessions require planning in the same way as preparation for delivering the content of the feedback.

During clinical placements, it is important to factor in opportunities for educators and students to discuss their expectations of the feedback process. The newly conceptualised feedback model presented in this chapter reinforces the importance of student self-evaluation during feedback sessions, and highlights that such reflection— *time to pause*—demands time, patience, intention and skill on behalf of the educator and the student. Educators' 'diagnostic tendency' in feedback often represents a translation from their clinical role where there is an emphasis on problem identification. This reinforces the need for formal upskilling of clinical educators in educational theory and practices to decrease a tendency to rely on extrapolation of knowledge and techniques from their clinical practice.

USING THEORIES TO DRIVE EDUCATION METHODS

Example: In providing feedback to students, it is important for the educator to ask the student to self-evaluate their performance, and to continue to probe for the learner's opinion if there is an attempt to deflect the self-analysis. This provision of opportunities for self-evaluation helps to diffuse the emotive responses to feedback frequently reported in the literature. It also encourages students to reflect on their practice and to make connections between their own performance and professional expectations and/or standards. Both student and educator are encouraged to collaborate to devise targeted strategies for improvement and, in subsequent feedback exchanges, there should be an explicit acknowledgement of changes in student performance.

Introduction

Feedback is key to learning, offering information on actual performance in relation to the intended goal of performance (Van de Ridder et al 2008, Askew 2000). In clinical education, feedback is used to identify students' strengths and weaknesses in performance, thereby promoting learning and behavioural change. Feedback can also provide motivation and has the potential to guide the student towards self-regulated practice (Molloy & Clarke 2005). Descriptors of effective feedback include that the message should be timely, based on first-hand data, focused on behaviours rather than learner qualities, and the provider and recipient should be positioned as allies during the interaction (Ende et al 1995, Latting 1992, Pendleton et al 1984). Although there is a growing body of literature devoted to feedback, distinct gaps remain in our understanding of the process and its impact on professional skill development (Nicol & Macfarlane-Dick 2006, Mugford et al 1991, Kluger & DeNisi 1996). This lack of clarity is largely due to the fact that feedback is a complex intervention that is dependent on the characteristics of the learning context, the source of the feedback, the individual recipient, and the message generated. It is the multidimensional nature of the process that makes the analysis of feedback interactions so challenging (Bucknall 2007, Ende et al 1995).

The lack of clarity and consensus in explanatory models of feedback can also be attributed to limited methodological approaches in the examination of feedback. To date, most of the feedback literature in health education is based on speculative assumptions rather than empirical studies. The paucity of pragmatic, real-world research into the context, conditions and ramifications of feedback in clinical education was the impetus for the research presented in this chapter.

This chapter has three aims. First, I will present the dominant conceptual ideas framing the delivery of feedback, most of which are derived from speculative or descriptive studies. Second, I will present the key aspects of an empirical study investigating face-to-face feedback in physiotherapy clinical education (Molloy 2006). Triangulation of perspectives underpins the methodological design of the research, where interpretation of the feedback process is provided by the students (self-report), clinical educators (self-report), and the researcher (observational data). Third, based on the empirical research findings, I will present recommendations for understanding and implementing effective feedback in clinical education that privileges the agentic and self-evaluative capacity of the learner.

Feedback literature

The dominant message in feedback literature is that feedback is problematic, both for the provider and the recipient (Henderson et al 2005, Ilgen & Davis 2000, Glover 2000, Ende et al 1995). Feedback has been described as 'hard to give, and hard to take'. In addition to the function of collecting data on student performance and synthesising this information into a meaningful and constructive message, the providers of feedback have to negotiate considerable social tensions in attempts to modify students' learning (Ende et al 1995). In the clinical education context, students are required to 'hear' the message, deconstruct it and reconstruct it in light of their current practice wisdom and, finally, act on the feedback. That is, students are expected to translate their clinical educator's advice into behaviour change. There is much written on the tendency for learners to react defensively to comment on their performance. Consequently much of the literature on feedback focuses on methods of 'gentle and diplomatic' feedback delivery.

Equally, clinical educators have reported feedback provision as challenging. Ende et al (1995) and Higgs et al (2004) suggest that clinical educators are required to balance a number of agendas when providing feedback, including protecting the patient, professional standards, and the self-esteem of the student. Educators have a responsibility to provide honest and accurate feedback, while balancing the social or affective needs of the junior member in the supervisory relationship. As reported by Higgs et al (2004): 'Giving feedback that preserves dignity and facilitates ongoing communication between the communication partners, but that also leads to behavioural change, is a challenge' (p 248).

The suggestion that feedback should be non-judgemental is widely supported (Ende 1983, Henry 1985, Hewson & Little 1998, Glover 2000). However Ende (1983) acknowledged an inherent danger in this 'non-judgemental approach'. He coined the concept of 'vanishing feedback' where the educator neglects to raise an issue for fear of eliciting a negative emotional reaction from the student. The student, in fearing a negative appraisal, may support and reinforce this educator avoidance. The message and the consequent potential for learning can be lost due to the perceived threat that 'feedback will have effects beyond its intent' (Ende 1983, p 778). This tension between acting with sensitivity and delivering with honesty presents a challenge to clinical educators. The literature provides clinical examples to demonstrate the potential damage of feedback on students' confidence, whether this be through the content of the message or the style of delivery (Cox & Ewan 1988, Stough & Emmer 1998). However clinical educators need to be aware of Ende's (1983) notion of 'vanishing feedback', where learning opportunities can be lost at the expense of attending to the student's emotional needs.

Another problematic feature of formal, face-to face feedback is that it has both learning and evaluative functions, and both students and educators have reported this tension in practice (Molloy & Clarke 2005, Glover 2000). Educators must position themselves to act as both mentor (providing constructive and encouraging support for learning) and assessor (providing judgement on how the learners' performance relates to practice norms). In drawing from the results of the feedback research, I argue for a shift in the feedback culture away from the didactic delivery of information from educator to student, towards a conversational model where students engage in the evaluative process. My key contention is that in order to achieve this change in culture, students need to develop self-evaluative capacities and need to be provided with space to exercise agency within the feedback interaction. Additionally, I argue for the educational advantages of upskilling students and educators to work within a solution-focused paradigm, instead of engaging in a largely diagnostic process that emphasises problem identification.

An empirical study of feedback

The aim of this research (Molloy 2006) was to observe and analyse the formal feedback interactions between student and clinical educator in physiotherapy clinical education, with the purpose of informing guidelines for effective practice. Formal feedback interactions are defined as the pre-arranged face-to-face sessions designed to discuss the student's performance. These formalised feedback sessions are embedded within the clinical education curricula in most health professions, and reflect the historical importance afforded to feedback as a learning tool.

The study used a mainly qualitative methodology and comprised three phases. A unique aspect of the methodology was the triangulation of three data sources, being self-report (interview), observation of practice (videotaping) and literature on best-practice feedback (Fig 8.1). In Phase 1, a questionnaire was designed and administered to elicit clinical educators' responses regarding current feedback practice, and their perceived affordances and constraints to providing effective feedback. The responses from this questionnaire informed the second phase of the project. Phase 2 involved the videotaping of eighteen formal feedback sessions and follow-up interviews with both students and educators. Phase 3 involved interviews with two key educators affiliated with the University of Melbourne to gain their opinions on the key themes to emerge from the study.

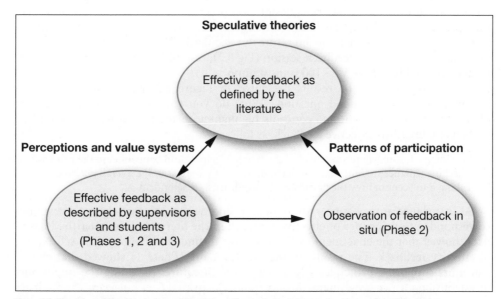

Figure 8.1 The interrelationship between literature, self-reported practice and patterns of participation

Few empirical studies have examined the feedback process in clinical education in situ, with the majority of the recommendations for effective practice based on theoretical constructs. The examination of the relationship between data sources is represented by double arrows in Figure 8.1.

The social practices and expectations implicit in the student–clinical educator interaction were a key focus of the study. Through data analysis, it became apparent that formal feedback constituted an ideal setting in which to: (1) examine the learning relationship between student and clinical educator, and (2) observe students' engagement with clinical practice and professional identity development. Harré & van Langenhove's (1999) Positioning Theory, as discussed in Chapter 4, was used as an analytical tool to examine the fine-grained social mechanics of the feedback sessions.

The research design enabled the tracking of students' progress from the start to the end of the clinical placement and therefore allowed for the examination of professional socialisation. The clinical education literature points to the complexity of the clinical environment and highlights students' growing independence and confidence as they are progressively socialised into the profession (Rose & Best 2005, Higgs et al 2004). Lave and Wenger (1991) described this phenomenon as 'legitimate peripheral participation' where individuals move from novice to expert status. Northedge (2003) also argued for a similar educational philosophy where students, through their participation in the discourse of the profession, are progressively socialised into a practice community.

There were three key findings from the research:
1 a disjunction between theory and practice
2 feedback enacted as a monologic process and
3 feedback as a vehicle for professional socialisation.

These themes are expanded upon below using supporting data, and a resultant model for the reconceptualisation of formal feedback in clinical education is presented.

Disjunction between theory and practice

Throughout the study, educators' descriptions of effective feedback practice were congruent with the espoused principles of 'best practice feedback' in the literature. For example, a striking characteristic of the questionnaire data was that clinical educators' responses closely mirrored the literature on feedback. When asked to rate factors important to an effective feedback session (Fig 8.2), respondents rated all factors except student age highly (where VAS 100 = most important).

In accordance with the results presented in Figure 8.2, participants' qualitative responses to the open-ended question, 'What do you view as the key characteristics of effective feedback?', reflected concepts highlighted in the literature. For example, a participant described 'effective feedback' as follows:

> Providing a forum where students feel they can participate and contribute to the process. Checking whether students have understood where they are at in the overall placement. Taking into account how the particular student learns. (Respondent 32)

At first glance, it may appear an innocuous finding that the participants' viewpoints corresponded to principles of effective feedback in the literature. However the Phase 2 data showed that the enactment of feedback was distinctly different to the self-reports of effective feedback. The results of the questionnaire (Phase 1) showed that clinical educators supported principles advocated in the literature, including the importance of establishing a two-way interaction in feedback. In practice, however, the feedback sessions did not represent two-way interactions. As stated by Kagan (1988), observational

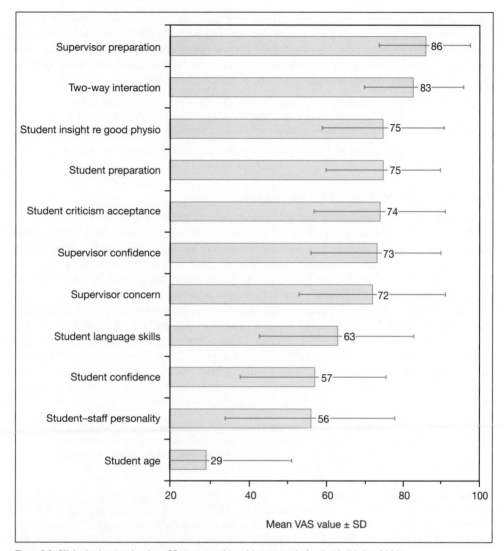

Figure 8.2 Clinical educators' rating of factors considered important in feedback (Molloy 2006)

methodology produces different results to self-report methodology. That is, what *we do* can be quite different to what *we say we do*, without necessarily reflecting an intention to deceive. The findings in this study reinforce the importance of triangulation of data sources in building an authentic picture of practice, and motivations for practice. The disjunction between theory and practice also calls for the detailed examination of factors that constrain educators and students from enacting their vision of ideal practice.

Formal feedback: a monologic culture

The key finding to emerge from the video-recording of the formal feedback encounters was that there was minimal input from the students in the sessions. Despite the educators providing students with an opportunity for self-evaluation at the start of most feedback sessions, students rarely took up this opportunity for engagement. In the eighteen videotaped interactions, there was no evidence of students collaborating to develop goals or strategies for improvement. On average, the feedback interactions lasted for 21 minutes, and the students' contribution accounted for less than two minutes of the 'conversation'. When interviewed, clinical educators acknowledged the one-way direction of the feedback sessions as indicated below:

> I felt that perhaps I talked too much, maybe just should have given her a bit more openness to talk throughout the session. Like she gave me some good comments at the end, but perhaps just could have paused a bit for her responses. (Clinical educator 1)

> Sometimes I catch myself and think you've been talking for a long time now. (Clinical educator 2)

Self-evaluation and tokenism

Consistent with clinical educators' self-reports about the importance of student self-analysis, the clinical educators observed did in fact provide opportunities for students to self-evaluate at the start and end of the sessions. The remarkable finding was that in most cases these invitations for self-analysis were not taken up by students. Rather the 'invitations' were judged by the researcher and two clinical educators in the sample as ritualistic, rather than a legitimate request for information.

The majority of clinical educators in the study acknowledged the uni-directional nature of feedback, and attributed this to time constraints, lack of trust in students' insight to formulate accurate self-evaluation, and complying with students' heightened sense of comfort by maintaining a didactic exchange. The impact of time as a pragmatic constraint to the practice of two-way feedback was raised repeatedly. It seems clear that a didactic style of feedback delivery is more time and resource efficient for clinical educators.

> We've all got time restraints so you know saying, 'What did you do well?' and then giving feedback, it all takes extra time, and that's an issue as well. And you know I find myself saying, 'Okay, what did you think?' and then hoping inside me that they'll be really quick about what they want to tell me. (Clinical educator, p 12)

In the nine case studies observed, only one clinical educator sought the in-depth opinion of her student in formal feedback. This clinical educator transgressed the characteristic feedback script, where clinical educators asked a tokenistic 'How do you think you are going?' followed by a clinical educator monologue. Instead, she further probed the student's self-analysis with follow-up questions, reducing the student's opportunity to escape with a superficial self-evaluative response. The educator asked for the student's opinion throughout the session and, additionally, validated the student's self-analysis with comments such as 'That is a good point that you've raised'.

The importance of clinical educator validation of students' self-analysis in feedback is supported by Frye et al (1997). In their study, Frye and colleagues found that clinical educators validated interns' self-assessment by either expressing agreement, or engaging the intern in a discussion that related to the issues which the intern voiced. In the research discussed in this chapter, clinical educators changed the direction of conversation swiftly away from students' self-evaluative comments, and there was seldom evidence of building on students' comments.

Both students and clinical educators expressed an understanding of the importance of two-way feedback. In sixteen out of eighteen videotaped sessions, clinical educators did provide invitations for student self-analysis, but the student responses in the feedback sessions indicated an expectation of tokenism. That is, students offered a brief account of their clinical experience, most often relating to their enjoyment of the clinical placement, rather than a commentary on learning or performance. The fact that clinical educators condoned this brief, or surface, response indicated that both students and clinical educators had shared expectations about the *meaning* of the self-evaluative invitation. The positioning dynamics of the educator and learner as described below offer a further explanation as to why students may be reticent to contribute to the feedback dialogue.

The clinical educator positioned as the diagnostician

There was a distinct 'positioning' of the clinical educator as the 'expert diagnostician', and the student as the 'attentive listener'. Both clinical educators and students were responsible for generating this style of feedback. Their values and beliefs about what their 'roles' embodied were reflected in their positioning practices, both in what they chose to say and chose not to say. The latter was the more informative feature in this study. In their interviews students commented on their lack of input into the feedback sessions, which often reflected their acquiescence to the expected social norms of the sessions rather than their level of knowledge.

This asymmetry in conversation observed between students and educators bears distinct resemblance to the asymmetry reported in patient–clinician conversations (Parry 2004). In a study of communicative interactions between physiotherapists and their patients, Parry (2004) found the observed conversations were entirely directed by the physiotherapist. Delany (2006) in a different study of physiotherapist–patient communication also noted the asymmetry in communication that constrained opportunities for patients to add to the conversation. The didactic nature of clinical communicative encounters is supported by Thornquist (1994). 'The relationship between therapist and patient is in principle asymmetric. The therapist's professional position enables her not only to define the problem and decide on the treatment, but also to control and define the encounter with the patient' (p 703).

The results from the feedback study suggested that students were equally responsible for creating this asymmetry in conversation. Students who praised their clinical educators most highly in feedback emerged from case studies where the sessions were shown to be most didactic in nature. Students cooperated with their clinical educator to position the clinical educator as the 'diagnostic expert', and did not contest their own positioning as the 'listener' in the interaction. This notion of 'complicity' was also raised in a study examining general practice consultations by Heath (1992). Heath's work contributes to the growing body of empirical research challenging the understanding that clinical authority, and the associated asymmetry in clinical interactions, is imposed on patients by clinicians. Consistent with the results of this study, Heath's research highlights that both patients and clinicians contribute to and in fact produce these features of 'unequal positioning' through their communicative actions.

It is too simplistic to frame clinical educators, with their superior knowledge bases and their inherent power over students in their role as assessors of student performance, as responsible for *imposing* this one-way culture of feedback. The study suggests that both students and clinical educators were jointly responsible for creating the one-way feedback culture observed, and that the communicative asymmetry represented an aspect of physiotherapy practice culture.

One clinical educator described the culture of feedback as an artefact of 'the physio way': 'Yes, I think that definitely goes on here [one-way feedback], no doubt. I think there's a lot of that that goes on because it's the physio way' (Clinical educator, p 12).

Clinical educators, as health practitioners, are conditioned to work within a biomedical paradigm where they are expected to assess patients, form a diagnosis of the presenting problem, and provide treatment for the problem. The way in which clinical educators provided feedback closely resembled this clinical positioning. Figure 8.3 compares the clinical and educational (giving feedback) demands of clinicians. The two practices share distinctly similar characteristics. The features of diagnosis, presenting data to support the diagnosis and providing treatment strategies, are commonly enacted in both educators' clinical practice and feedback practice.

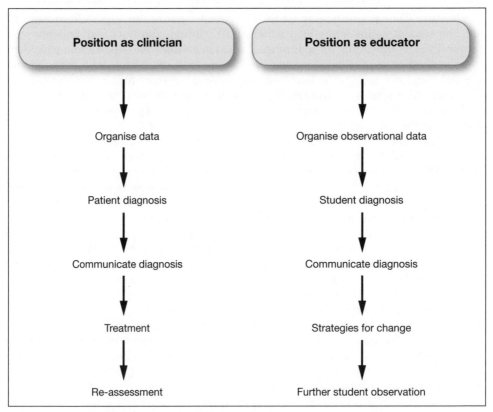

Figure 8.3 Juxtaposing clinical practice and clinical educator positions

A descriptive study by Latting (1992) suggested that clinical educators have a tendency to adopt a diagnostic role in feedback as an extrapolation from their clinical knowledge paradigm. Bourdieu's (1977) work on Habitus also reports a similar tendency for humans to extrapolate a framework of values, behaviours and skills from one setting to another discreet setting. Clinically trained clinical educators who have developed skills in assessing the underlying causes of behaviour may be especially prone to offer their interpretations of a subordinate's behaviour (Latting 1992, p 426).

One concern relating to the clinical educator positioned as the 'diagnostician' is that the biomedical clinical model emphasises *deficit*. That is, when a health practitioner analyses a patient's gait pattern, there is a tendency to search for the deficit in movement and hypothesise the reasons for the problem, rather than searching for a strength in the movement pattern. In the feedback sessions observed, such a focus on students' deficits was *not* apparent. However the literature on feedback in the health professions has identified that clinical educators can neglect to provide a balance of corrective and reinforcing comments (Bucknall 2007, Frye et al 1997, Ende et al 1995).

Clinical educators did not *impose* a didactic, authoritarian manner upon students. Students were also active in perpetuating these mutually created and accepted positions within the feedback culture. They viewed clinical educators as diagnosticians with superior content knowledge, experiential knowledge and institutional knowledge, and invited their diagnostic approach to the feedback sessions. The data indicate that students' reticence to provide input into their feedback session was attributable to factors including: self-analysis required more effort; it provided a site for potential loss of face should student and clinical educator express disparate opinions; and that students were sensitive to the need to maintain social harmony within the sessions. This concern for social cohesion (or lack of conflict) was compounded by the fact that clinical educators were acting as assessors.

> We don't do a lot of that [self-evaluation] is the short answer. And the reason is that a lot of the time we found that students aren't comfortable with that. So because they're not comfortable with that, and it's a lot quicker getting through it this way, we don't do it. (Clinical educator, p 14)

Table 8.1 summarises the educator and student-centred factors that may constrain a two-way feedback process.

EDUCATOR FACTORS	STUDENT FACTORS
• Clinical educator may be limited in time (balancing patient load, administration load and student load) • Clinical educator may not be skilled in facilitating students' self-evaluation • Clinician adherence to historical 'apprenticeship models' of clinical education practice • Clinician tendency to 'diagnose' and 'fix' rather than engage in collaborative decision making (transference from clinical paradigm)	• Student reticence to evaluate their own performance through fear of being wrong (saving face) • Student 'positioning' of the educator as content–practice expert • Student concern in challenging educator's view due to reasons of power–hierarchy • Student perfectionism and concern for assessment rather than learning

Table 8.1 Factors constraining two-way feedback practice

Feedback as a vehicle for professional socialisation

The feedback literature in health education focuses on how to provide students with information to improve *performance*. This study highlighted a further role that feedback might play: that of providing a 'safe' forum removed from the immediate demands of patient care to enculturate students into the profession. In feedback sessions, educators provided students with insight into implicit and explicit aspects of the curriculum, and disclosed aspects of their own clinical practice, including difficulties they had experienced. Such self-disclosure positioned the students as junior colleagues and afforded them more status as members of the profession rather than as peripheral participants.

Observation of the feedback sessions revealed that 'teaching' beyond direct feedback on students' performance constituted a large part of the feedback sessions. This form of enculturation included unpacking or explaining the meanings of assessment criteria and explanations for why physiotherapists act in certain ways, for example historical, institutional and hierarchical influences. An example of this teaching about the profession is shown below. In this example, the clinical educator provided information beyond 'you need to write more detailed notes'.

> Clinical educator: Like the progress notes you wrote today, technically they were fine but they were very brief. There could have been a whole lot more qualification in them.
>
> Student: Yep.
>
> Clinical educator: Because that's our only opportunity as physios to impart our assessment and what we're doing to the rest of the team. And if the medical staff come along and read those notes, they're going to be none the wiser. They are not going to understand why the patient needs follow-up after discharge. (Clinical educator)

In the sessions, clinical educators provided aspects of knowledge that were not necessarily part of the overt, academic curriculum. Frye et al's (1997) study on feedback conversations in medical education similarly demonstrated that clinical educators 'used various instructional techniques that went beyond simple performance assessment' (p 217). With the exception of findings from this study, the feedback literature focuses on the value of feedback in changing performance. The literature does not attend to the educators' ability to use feedback as a way to teach the student about the community of knowledge they are entering. The research data from this study suggests that clinical educators used formal feedback sessions as a forum to communicate explicit and implicit characteristics of the curriculum, along with characteristics of their own practice (self-disclosure).

Clinical educator self-disclosure

The literature on professional socialisation emphasises that it is through relationships, and most often those between student and educator, that professional socialisation occurs (Cox & Ewan 1988, McAllister et al 1997). Through sharing their knowledge, clinical educators can encourage students to develop expectations of themselves and others within the clinical context. Self-disclosure can serve a number of functions, including empathy and encouragement. In the example below, the clinical educator confessed that she too had experienced difficulty with a skill (auscultation). The clinical educator *normalised* the students' difficulty with the skill, and implied through her own disclosure that it improves with time. It may also be argued that the educator's own confession of her performance deficit (ability to give up face), may have encouraged the student to follow suit. That is, she modelled that it was acceptable to expose her vulnerabilities in learning and practice through conversation with peers.

> Just with auscultation, in terms of being unsure with what you're hearing. We were all in that boat. [Joint laughter.] We were all thinking 'are they crackles that I'm hearing or just …', so it's just more practice listening on patients, brothers, sisters, colleagues. And you know, if you're listening to patients and you're not sure what you're hearing, just ask us and we'll pop the stethoscope on and listen to what you're hearing. (Clinical educator, p 4)

Hargie et al (1981) and Brown (1993) previously recognised that experts' self-disclosure helped to reduce power asymmetry and promote open communication in educational relationships. Formal feedback provides one of the only opportunities for a face-to-face student–educator interaction in a private setting removed from patients, peers and other health professionals. In this setting, students are well positioned to communicate their own construction of self as related to expected performance (self-evaluation) as well as their constructions of professional practice.

Time to pause: a reconceptualisation of feedback

The data in this study highlight that feedback practice deviates considerably from principles of 'best practice' highlighted in the literature and advocated by participants. Considering that both students and clinical educators reported that they were comfortable with the positioning of the clinical educator as the authority in feedback (diagnostician), and that clinical educators acknowledged that didactic communication was a more efficient process, is there in fact an argument for the value of two-way feedback?

To answer this question it is important to return to adult learning literature which advocates that students' ability to self-evaluate their own performance is a key skill required for lifelong learning (McAllister et al 1997, Biggs 1993, Mezirow 1991, Higgs 1992, Barrows 1986). The model presented in Figure 8.4 reconceptualises feedback practice and recognises that feedback provides functions other than facilitating the improvement of clinical performance alone. The deviations in best practice feedback observed in the study highlight opportunities to develop a broader role for feedback in clinical education.

The research demonstrates that both educators and students are reluctant to engage in a two-way feedback interaction. Instead they position themselves within 'comfort zones' (that have been historically established and mutually understood) of the 'expert diagnositician' and 'passive recipient'. While this uptake and enactment of roles is understandable given time constraints and historical expectations of the role of teacher and learner, it points to the need for a more inclusive and ambitious view of what feedback is capable of achieving. In this final section of this chapter, I present a model to reconceptualise feedback (Fig 8.4) that explicitly elevates self-evaluation and professional socialisation as components and outcomes of a collaborative feedback process.

Figure 8.4 represents the multiple functions of feedback as ways to improve (1) students' clinical skills (the focus of feedback literature), (2) students' self-evaluative skills, and (3) students' smooth entry into the discourse of the professional community. The bold arrow on the left-hand side represents the pathway emphasised in the feedback literature. This function was highlighted as the key purpose of feedback by students and clinical educators in this study. The additional two arrows have derived from this research, and signal that the process of developing self-evaluative and professional engagement skills through feedback are underprivileged both in the current enactment of feedback sessions and in the relevant literature.

This model challenges existing concepts of feedback presented in health professional education. Although student self-evaluation is advocated as a strategy to improve the effectiveness of feedback, it is not seen as an outcome of effective feedback. I am proposing that formal feedback sessions are an ideal forum for clinical educators to model evaluative processes to students and to scaffold students' own development of self-evaluative skills. A culture of monologic feedback, where clinical educators are positioned as diagnosticians, does not afford students with opportunities to build on these reflective practice skills.

The other advantage of a two-way conversation is that it allows participants an opportunity to check for shared understanding of content. The education literature warns against making assumptions about shared understanding in conversation; that is, that the content delivered by one party is interpreted in the same way by the receiver (McAllister et al 1997).

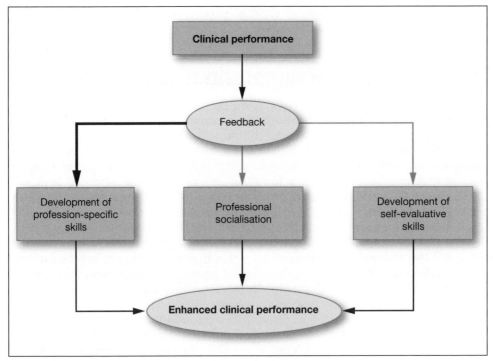

Figure 8.4 Reconceptualisation of the functions of feedback (Molloy 2006)

Practical recommendations for implementing feedback

The major finding to emerge from the study was that despite intentions to create a two-way feedback process, clinical educators and students conspired to produce a one-way feedback culture. Some of the constraints (such as perceived tensions between affect and performance) were viewed as artefacts of the feedback rhetoric, rather than as immovable and innate features of the process. Likewise, the tendency for clinical educators to diagnose and fix students, rather than engaging in collaborative diagnosis and decision making, was viewed as an artefact of clinical practice culture. By taking into account the re-conceptualised functions of feedback, the following recommendations are made to improve the practice of feedback in clinical education. The education of both students and clinical educators on the importance of feedback in learning, including the provision of guidelines for engaging in 'effective' practice, is paramount. Ideally students should be encouraged to participate in an 'evaluative community of practice' early in their orientation to the university setting that will equip them with the necessary skills to effectively negotiate a complex and changing healthcare environment.

Recommendation 1 Provide explicit teaching on principles of effective feedback early in the academic curriculum

The skills of giving and receiving feedback are not only relevant to students' clinical learning at the undergraduate level, but are lifelong skills that will help them to refine and develop their clinical practice. It can also be argued that the ability to provide patients with feedback, for example on their newly acquired movement or on their change of lifestyle, is central to healthcare practice (Henderson et al 2005).

It is recommended that feedback be taught explicitly as a skill in the academic curriculum in the health professions. That is, prior to students' embarking on their clinical placements, they are exposed to both theoretical and practical applications of feedback. It is important that students understand the theoretical underpinnings of effective feedback practice, including the characteristics and philosophy of student-centred learning, coupled with ongoing opportunities to practise feedback skills. 'What individuals accomplish with the concept of feedback and what they perceive its strengths and limitations to be depend on the sources of their understandings of it' (Richardson 2004, p 1).

The results of this study, and the rhetoric in the health education literature (Cupit 1988, Higgs 1992, Bogo 1993, Kilminster & Jolly 2000) demonstrate that students' entry into the domain of clinical education is challenging. Students need to be equipped with the skills to engage in face-to-face feedback prior to engaging in the complex clinical education program. In clinical education, students are confronted with new institutional and professional demands, and must negotiate the expectations of feedback encounters. If students are cognisant of the underpinning purposes of feedback, and are experienced and confident in dealing with face-to-face feedback exchanges, the culture of feedback may be substantially different.

The teaching of feedback philosophy and skills should be integrated early into undergraduate curricula to ensure that students build progressive mastery in these skills. Henderson et al (2005) emphasise the need for early opportunities in skill development so that evaluative processes are framed as habit, rather than feared encounters. 'We are concerned with how to develop a work culture into which is built the learning and application of the skills required for giving and receiving both positive and negative feedback, regardless of the position of colleagues in the hierarchy, such that the use of these skills becomes second nature and not an act of bravery' (p 6).

It is equally important that clinical educators are provided with adequate education on the philosophy and skills underpinning the giving and receiving of feedback (Palinscar (1998). Further educational sessions that focus on enactment of feedback skills, including developing strategies for performance change, should be made available to clinical educators.

Ende (1983) devised feedback guidelines that still have relevancy in contemporary clinical education settings. Pendleton et al (1984) and Silverman et al (1996) have also devised feedback models with similar properties to Ende's model. These guidelines, which emphasise the importance of focusing on observed behaviours and establishing goals for performance improvement, may be taught explicitly to both educators and students.

Table 8.2 is derived from the research data and presents a framework for clinical educators and students to use to appraise their role and practice in feedback. This reflection on feedback practice requires that the educator 'pause' and consider the mechanics of their message delivery and its potential effect on student learning. The 'power of the pause' is referred to in the literature on feedback (Ende et al 1995, Neville & French 1991), namely as a way of providing the student with space to self-evaluate their performance. In support of Schön's (1987) reflection 'on' and 'in' practice, I argue that along with pausing during feedback practice, clinical educators need to regularly pause after providing feedback to evaluate the educational opportunities and outcomes they have co-constructed with the student.

Student agency, power symmetry, message content, and clear strategies for improvement are emphasised in the analytical framework.

DIMENSIONS TO CONSIDER WHEN PROVIDING FEEDBACK	AS THE EDUCATOR, ASK YOURSELF …
Interaction (one- versus two-way conversation, clinical educator skill in facilitating self-analysis)	Who did most of the talking?
Power and positioning dynamics (verbal content and body language)	How did I position myself in relation to the student? Did I use inclusive and encouraging language?
Clinical educator responsiveness to the student's comments	How did I respond to the student's questions and comments?
Content (balance of positive and negative comments)	What was the focus of my comments: deficits or strengths?
Supporting data (provision of examples of *behaviour*)	What specific behaviour did I refer to?
Strategies for improvement (using solution-focused framework)	What concrete strategy did I suggest that was achievable for the student? Are my comments based in the past, present or future?
Summarising and clarification for shared meaning	Did I check that the student shared or understood my analysis?

Table 8.2 Framework for analysis of feedback (Molloy 2006)

Recommendation 2 Encourage student self-evaluation: pauses and questions
The results from this study indicate that both students and clinical educators need to take responsibility to produce a dialogic form of feedback. It could be argued, however, that clinical educators as the party with more inherent power in the relationship have a heightened responsibility to shape the feedback sessions in a way that encourages student input.

This function of feedback to encourage students' development of self-analytical skills needs to be made explicit to learners and clinical educators. Clinical educators need to better scaffold students' self-evaluative practices with the use of questions beyond the superficial 'How are you finding the placement?' A series of questions, such as those shown below, are more likely to challenge students to reflect on their practice and communicate their analysis. This style of questioning encourages students to engage in 'story-telling', a technique recommended by Frye et al (1997) and Williams & Wilkins (1999); for example:

- Can you tell me how you went in your treatment with Mrs X?
- What do you think you did well?
- What do you think you could improve next time?
- Can you summarise the key points that you have gained from today's feedback session?

Along with questioning, another key technique recommended in feedback is use of 'the pause'. Ende et al (1995) and Neville & French (1991) suggested that clinical educators' use of pausing as an 'opportunity space' allowed the student to reflect on and reframe their responses.

Recommendation 3 Encourage students to seek feedback from alternative sources to the clinical educator
Central to the argument for improvement of feedback practice in clinical education is that students need to learn to value the giving and receiving of feedback as a lifelong skill. Learners need to be positioned as responsible for seeking feedback to help improve their

performance, and should look to multiple sources of feedback to inform the construction of their own practice. Acknowledgment that feedback can come from different sources (including self) may ease the conception that feedback is something inflicted on students by clinical educators. It may also help students to recognise the subjective nature of feedback; that is, the clinical educator is providing their own interpretation of student performance, and this interpretation may be different from the student's or patient's understanding of the encounter. The application of multi-source or '360 degree' feedback is gathering momentum in health education, particularly in the postgraduate and ongoing professional development arenas (Ilgen & Davis 2000, Richardson 2004, Kluger & DeNisi 1996).

There is ample literature on the value of peer feedback and peer evaluation in health education (Gandy & Jensen 1992, McAllister et al 1997, Vuorinen et al 2000). The advantage of peer feedback is that the tensions of assessment are removed. The results of the Molloy (2006) study suggested that clinical educators' dual roles as both assessor and mentor may have inhibited the students' honesty and active contribution in the feedback sessions. It may be that staff need to facilitate peer learning by establishing informal learning groups within the clinical schools, and encourage regular peer-to-peer feedback. One strategy for addressing this student reticence to discuss feedback with peers would be to formalise face-to-face peer feedback encounters.

Recommendation 4 A solution-focused approach to learning

Both educators and students report difficulty in providing and receiving constructive feedback due to the emotive element implicit in performance appraisal (Molloy 2006, Frye et al 1997, Ende et al 1995). A key strategy to address this 'tension' is to focus on strategies for change, rather than labouring on the identified deficits in learner performance. This focus on strategy development for behavioural change is a key tenet in Ende's (1983) feedback model and Molloy's (2006) feedback framework (see Table 8.2).

Devlin (2003) highlights a model for learning called solution-focused brief therapy (SFBT), extrapolated from the psychology domain (Berg & Miller 1992, Davis & Osborn 2000). The central premises of the SFBT model are described in Table 8.3, and reflect the aims of feedback described in this chapter. The model is based on a learner-centred approach to education where the learner is committed to the goals of feedback. There is a 'subtle but underpinning' expectation of improvement, which is reflected in the language of the feedback provider. The process of feedback is orientated towards the future, that is change, rather than the reconstruction of past events. In my study, students' reported frustration in being 'diagnosed' as incompetent early in the clinical rotation, and that the example of poor performance continued to be raised in subsequent feedback sessions. The SFBT model favours a 'glass half-full' philosophy with a focus on the generation of solutions rather than problem identification.

Conclusion

The research presented in this chapter highlights the tendency for clinical educators to reside in their clinical practice frame of comfort. Clinical educators justified their didactic delivery of feedback and focus on analysis of deficit based on their familiarity with the clinical paradigm, that is 'the physio way'. The solution-focused model of learning, extrapolated from the psychology literature, departs from the emphasis on 'problem-identification' and privileges the formation of attainable solutions. Embedded in the

KEY PREMISES OF SOLUTION-FOCUSED PRACTICE	FURTHER EXPLANATION
1 The goal of the intervention is determined by the learner, based on their context, resources and strengths	The student 'should' have insight into what constitutes workable solutions in the clinical education environment. However students early in their clinical placements may find devising realistic solutions more challenging, and the educator may need to help formulate and refine solutions.
2 Change is viewed as inevitable and improvement as likely	Through the skilled use of language, discussions are orientated to the present and future, not the past. This orientation to present and future is essential for the commitment to encouraging change. Students commonly resent clinicians repeatedly referring to a past action (see Ch 9 'Halo and devil effect'), particularly if they have demonstrated consequent behaviour change. The language also implies inevitability of behaviour change, e.g. change is couched in terms of 'when' not 'if'.
3 Looking for exceptions to problems	This is a case of reverse engineering 'problems', i.e. looking for problems and 'non-problems'. Educators and students look for examples of clinical practice when the problem does not occur, as it is in these 'exceptions' that the roots of solutions are found.
4 Interventions should be strategically chosen, employed and re-assessed	Strategies for behaviour change should be recognisable and attainable. If a chosen strategy is working, its use should be continued or increased. If not working, the approach needs to be changed. This philosophy of 'application of intervention and re-assessment for change' is a key tenet in clinical healthcare practice and should be familiar to clinical educators and students.

Table 8.3 Key tenets of solution-focused practice

model is a form of 'positioning' where the educator positions the learner as capable and on the way to achieving the new practice goals. Additionally, by reverse engineering the concept of 'problem', students and educators can look for examples of effective student practice ('non-problems') in order to formulate solutions.

Both students and clinical educators are complicit in shaping the feedback process and its impact on learning. Therefore a change in feedback practice demands that both parties assume responsibility within the interaction. The research has highlighted constraints to students' engagement in the formal feedback sessions, and it is hoped the suggested recommendations may encourage a shift in the culture of feedback towards that of a conversation. It is through conversations that students develop shared meanings and contribute to the discourse of the profession.

References

Askew S 2000 Feedback for learning. Routledge Falmer, London

Barrows H 1986 A Taxonomy of problem-based learning methods. Medical Education 20:481–486

Berg I, Miller S 1992 Working with the problem drinker: a solution-focused approach. Norton, New York

Biggs J 1993 From theory to practice: a cognitive systems approach. Higher Education and Research Development 12:73–85

Bogo M 1993 The student/field instructor relationship: the critical factor in field education. The Clinical Educator 11:23–36

Bourdieu P 1977 Outline of a theory of practice. Cambridge University Press, UK

Brown G 1993 Accounting for power: nurse teachers' and students' perceptions of power in their relationship. Nurse Education Today 13:111–120

Bucknall T 2007 Carrots, sticks and sermons: is feedback the answer to changing clinicians' behaviour? Worldviews on Evidence-based Nursing 103:1–2

Cox R, Ewan C 1988 The medical teacher, 2nd edn. Churchill Livingstone, Melbourne, p 9–14

Cupit R 1988 Student stress: an approach to coping at the interface between preclinical and clinical education. Australian Journal of Education 34:215–219

Davis T, Osborn C 2000 The solution-focused school counselor. Taylor & Francis, Philadelphia

Delany C 2006 Informed consent: ethical theory, legal obligations and the physiotherapy clinical encounter. Centre for the Study of Health in Society. University of Melbourne, Melbourne

Devlin M 2003 A solution-focused model for improving individual university teaching. International Journal for Academic Development 8:77–89

Ende J 1983 Feedback in clinical medical education. Journal of American Medical Association 250:777–781

Ende J, Pomerantz A, Erickson F 1995 Preceptors' strategies for correcting residents in an ambulatory care medicine setting: a qualitative analysis. Academic Medicine 70, 224–229

Frye A, Hollingsworth M, Wymer A, Hinds A 1997 A qualitative study of faculty techniques for giving feedback to interns following an observed standardised patient encounter. In: Scherpbier A, van der Vleuten C, Rethans J, van der Steeg A (eds) Advances in medical Education. Kluwer Academic Publishers, Dordrecht, p 216–219

Gandy J, Jensen G 1992 Group work and reflective practicums in physical therapy education: models for professional behavior development. Journal of Physical Therapy Education 6(1):6–10

Glover P 2000 'Feedback. I listened, reflected and utilised': third year nursing students' perceptions and use of feedback in the clinical setting. International Journal of Nursing Practice 6:247–250

Hargie O, Saunders C, Dickson D 1981 Social skills in interpersonal communication. Croom Helm, Beckenham, Kent

Harré R, van Langenhove L 1999 Positioning theory. Blackwell, Oxford

Heath C 1992 The delivery and reception of diagnosis in the general practice consultation. In: Drew P, Heritage J (eds) Talk at work-interaction in institutional settings. Cambridge University Press, UK

Henderson P, Ferguson-Smith A, Johnson M 2005 Developing essential professional skills: a framework for teaching and learning about feedback. BMC Medical Education 5:1–6

Henry J 1985 Using feedback and evaluation effectively in clinical supervision. Physical Therapy 65:354–357

Hewson M, Little M 1998 Giving feedback in medical education. Journal of General Internal Medicine 13:111–117

Higgs J 1992 Managing clinical education: the educator–manager and the self-directed learner. Physical Therapy 78:822–828

Higgs J, Richardson B, Abrandt Dahlgren M 2004 Developing practice knowledge for health professionals. Butterworth-Heinemann, Edinburgh

Igen D, Davis A 2000 Bearing bad news: reactions to negative performance feedback. Applied Psychology: An International Review 49:550–565

Kagan D 1988 Research on the supervision of counsellors- and teachers-in-training: Linking two bodies of literature. Review of Educational Research 58:1–24

Kilminster S, Jolly B 2000 Effective supervision in clinical practice settings: a literature review. Medical Education 34:827–840

Kluger A, DeNisi A 1996 The effects of feedback interventions on performance: a historical review, a meta-analysis and a preliminary feedback intervention theory. Psychological Bull 119:254–284

Latting J 1992 Giving corrective feedback: a decisional analysis. Social Work 37:424–430

Lave J, Wenger E 1991 Situated learning: legitimate peripheral participation. Cambridge University Press, UK

McAllister L, Lincoln M, McLeod S, Maloney D 1997 Facilitating learning in clinical settings. Nelson Thornes, London

Mezirow J 1991 Transformative dimensions of adult learning. Jossey-Bass, San Francisco

Molloy E 2006 Insights into the formal feedback culture in physiotherapy clinical education. School of Physiotherapy and Department of Education, University of Melbourne, Melbourne

Molloy E, Clarke D 2005 The positioning of physiotherapy students and clinical educators in feedback sessions. Focus on Health Professional Education: A Multi-disciplinary Journal 7:79–90

Mugford M, Banfiedl R, O'Hanlon M 1991 Effects of feedback information on clinical practice: A review. British Medical Journal 303:398–402

Neville S, French S 1991 Clinical education: students' and clinical tutors' views. Physiotherapy 77:351–354

Nicol D, Macfarlane-Dick D 2006 Formative assessment and self-regulated learning: a model and seven principles of good feedback practice. Studies in Higher Education 31:199–218

Northedge A 2003 Enabling participation in academic discourse. Teaching in Higher Education 8:169–180

Palinscar A 1998 Social constructivist perspectives on teaching and learning. Annual Review of Psychology 49:345–375

Parry R 2004 Communication during goal-setting in physiotherapy treatment sessions. Clinical Rehabilitation 18:668–682

Pendleton D, Schofield T, Tate P, Havelock P 1984 The consultation: an approach to learning and teaching. Oxford University Press, Oxford

Richardson B 2004 Feedback. Academic Emergency Medicine 11:1–5

Rose M, Best D 2005 Transforming practice through clinical education, professional supervision and mentoring. Elzevier, Edinburgh

Schön D 1987 Educating the reflective practitioner. Jossey-Bass, London

Silverman J, Kurtz S, Draper J 1996 The Calgary–Cambridge approach to communication skills teaching: agenda-led, outcome-based analysis of the conversation. Education in General Practice 7:288–299

Stough L, Emmer E 1998 Teachers' emotions and test feedback. Qualitative Studies in Education 11:341–361

Thornquist E 1994 Profession and life—separate worlds. Social Science and Medicine 39:701–713

van de Ridder M, Stokking K, McGaghie W, Olle T 2008 What is feedback in clinical education? Medical Education 42:189–197

Vuorinen R, Tarkka MT, Meretoja R 2000 Peer evaluation in nurses' professional development: a pilot study to investigate the issues. Journal of Clinical Nursing 9:273–281

Williams RM, Wilkins S 1999 The use of reflective summary writing as a method of obtaining student feedback about entering physical therapy practice. Journal of Physical Therapy Education 13:28–33

CHAPTER 9

Assessment in clinical education

Jenny Keating, Megan Dalton and Megan Davidson

THEORIES

The key theoretical perspectives that underscore this chapter about performance-based assessment are *sociocultural* theories of learning. These theories frame learning and assessment of learning as a process of participation in activities that are situated in a range of clinically based social and cultural contexts. In addition, theories that relate to *critical reflection* are used to frame the importance of clinical educators demonstrating a level of reflexivity so that they are open to recognising their own cognitive bias or premature decision making when assessing students.

USING THEORIES TO INFORM CURRICULUM DESIGN AND RESEARCH

When designing assessment tasks within clinical education curricula, it is important to distinguish between performance-based assessment and competency-based assessment (measuring what is done in testing situations). Using sociocultural theories to frame the way students learn means acknowledging the learner is dealing with complexity, uncertainty, and continual changes in service provision ethos and practice. On the basis of this layered and more nuanced recognition, it is argued that the best way to gather a reliable and valid representation of students' skills in clinical practice is via longitudinal monitoring of students' performance. Such longitudinal assessment encourages observation of practice in a range of learning circumstances. In this way, assessment is viewed as an opportunity for educators to provide learners with clear, practical and relevant information and direction, and to help learners develop skills of self-evaluation and self-regulation.

USING THEORIES TO DRIVE EDUCATION METHODS

Example: The Assessment of Physiotherapy Practice (APP) is presented as a practical example of developing clear criteria that can be linked to explicit and detailed performance indicators. These performance indicators have been developed to reduce assessor bias and to provide students with clear practice goals. Such detailed and transparent expectations grounded in the realities of students' learning experiences assist them to 'unpack' and make sense of their professional discourse and clinical practice. The assessment tool encourages students to reflect on their own performance in relation to the explicit behavioural descriptions.

Introduction

The aim of this chapter is to introduce key concepts and strategies in assessment of clinical practice for health practitioner students. We define the role of and rationale for assessment of clinical skills, and present an empirically developed assessment instrument, Assessment of Physiotherapy Practice (APP), for use in clinical education.

Assessment drives learning

Assessment should impact positively on future learning (van der Vleuten 1996). It provides targets that focus and drive the depth and direction of learning for students. For educators, assessment provides opportunities for feedback to students on current performance, and enables the development of specific strategies to improve performance and achieve learning outcomes. Assessment targets include the foundation knowledge of health sciences, clinical skills and important domains of practice such as habits of reflection and professional behaviour, interpersonal skills, commitment to lifelong learning, and integration of relevant and current knowledge into practice (Epstein 2007, Epstein & Hundert 2002).

Students are directed to skill acquisition using well-constructed learning objectives. Quality assessment should be aligned with, and guide the achievement of, these objectives. In the clinical delivery of heath services, this presents the challenge of assessing a large number of learning objectives covering a broad spectrum of professional practices. Stakeholders with a vested interest in ensuring the quality of practice provided by health professionals might be particularly interested in the design of student assessment. Assessment that is continuously reviewed and refined, addressing student and stakeholder feedback and evaluation, can remain aligned with changing expectations of graduate ability. In some health professions, for example physiotherapy, students graduate with primary contact practitioner status. It is therefore essential that assessment identifies students as competent across the required spectrum of professional practice.

Why assess?

Assessment in the health sciences serves many purposes, as shown in Box 9.1.

Methods used for assessing professional competence

In 1990 psychologist George Miller proposed a pyramid of hierarchy in the assessment of clinical competence. From lowest to highest, the levels were defined as knows, knows how (competence), shows how (performance), and does (action) (Fig 9.1).

BOX 9.1 The purpose of assessment in health sciences

The purpose of assessment is to:
- drive student learning
- certify the competence of future practitioners
- direct attention to the competencies specified by accrediting or qualifying bodies
- specify the levels of knowledge or skill required for entry into different categories of practitioner
- identify underperformance and enable targeted remediation
- discriminate among candidates for awards, scholarships, advanced training or specialisation.

Assessment of the highest level of 'action' involves identifying acceptable performance during typical practice. Rethans et al (2002) draw a clear distinction between (1) competency-based assessments or measuring what is done in testing situations, and (2) performance-based assessments, measuring what is done in practice. Important differences between the two are that competency assesses what is known and uses known conditions, equipment and methods, but performance in practice requires dealing with emotional states, uncertainty, complex circumstances and ongoing changes in systems of service provision and expectations. Performance-based assessments are also predicated on sociocultural theories of learning in which learning is understood as a process of participation in activities situated in appropriate social and cultural contexts (Lave & Wenger 1991). Wass et al (2001) called assessment of the pyramid apex (Fig 9.1) the 'does', as 'the international challenge of the century for all involved in clinical competence testing' (p 948). This chapter will focus on methods of performance assessment.

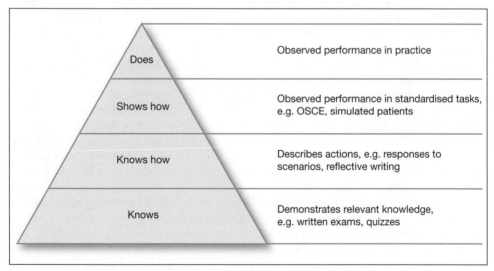

Figure 9.1 Miller's (1990) triangle applied to education of health professional students

Professional education programs typically assess across all levels of clinical competence and include direct assessment of clinical practice. It is assumed that observed practice in the operational context is an indicator of likely professional performance (Wiggins 1989, p 711). The assessment of 'does' is required for certifying fitness to practice. Professional practice necessitates understanding and dealing with highly variable circumstances, and assessment is therefore difficult to standardise across students (Rethans et al 2002). A proposed solution to this complexity is to monitor students over a sufficiently long period of time to enable observation of practice in a range of circumstances and across a spectrum of patient types and needs. This has been argued as superior to one-off 'exit style' examinations (van der Vleuten 2000). It also enables assessment to encompass local contexts, cultures and workplaces within which learners must demonstrate competence (see Ch 3). Longitudinal monitoring is a form of longitudinal assessment that guides the evolution of professional habits such as reflective practices and ongoing learning. Longitudinal assessment can be subtle and continuous or intermittent and structured.

Formative and summative assessment

In broad terms, assessment can be applied in two ways: to determine competence and to guide skill development. Occasions that provide feedback on performance but are not graded (formative assessment) enable students to attempt the task without the confounding influence of fear of failing. Formative assessment outcomes guide future learning, provide reassurance, promote reflection and shape values (Epstein 2007, Molloy 2006). However it needs to be frequent and constructive (Boud 1995, Epstein 2007). Students need regular, clear and behaviourally specific feedback based on the educator's assessment of their performance in order to devise and implement strategies to effect positive change.

Other important elements of formative assessment are that it should mimic graded (summative) assessment to familiarise the student with both the expected performance and their current skill levels, and to aid in devising a path for improving performance. When formative assessment mimics summative assessment, anxieties associated with summative assessment can be reduced through clarification of desired performance. Formative assessment provides a vehicle for the important work of gathering evidence of student learning in a way that supports the learning process (Masters 1999, p 20). As described in Chapter 8, learning through feedback, as a form of formative assessment, enables constructive discussion about student practices in a supportive environment where strategies to decrease anxiety and facilitate enquiry are deliberately introduced. These elements are important for students at all levels of achievement and are particularly important when the student is in danger of failing summative assessments. Learning through interaction and discussion is enhanced because formative assessment is less likely to invite a defensive reaction about student ability, as might occur in summative assessment where the effect on a student's grade can create anxiety.

A further important element is the timing of formative assessment. Ideally it should be provided to enable adequate opportunity for skill development prior to summative assessment so as to further reduce associated anxiety and enable the planning of effective strategies that can be tested and modified to achieve learning goals. An important outcome of formative assessment is documentation of evidence of what was discussed so that all parties are very clear about the behaviours that would signal improved performance. Educators and students can crystallise the elements in performance that require attention and convert these to achievable goals.

Current practice in assessment of competency in allied health professions

Despite extensive literature on the issues underlying the assessment of clinical competence, the choice of assessment approach is typically influenced by historical precedents and the personal experiences of assessors, rather than known psychometric properties of assessment instruments (Newble et al 1994). Given the high stakes of undergraduate summative assessments of clinical competence, assessment procedures should not only be feasible and practical but also demonstrate sufficient reliability and validity for the purpose (Epstein & Hundert 2002, Roberts et al 2006, Wass et al 2001). Standardisation of clinical performance may be confounded by difficulties associated with unavoidable variations in test items, assessors, patients and examination procedures (Roberts et al 2006). Specific difficulties have been reported in relation to:

- the complexity and variety of clinical tasks including patient mix, complexity and numbers of patients (Petrusa 2002)
- the complexity and variety of clinical contexts and service delivery methods (Kurth et al 2001, Oldmeadow 1996, Struber 2004)
- the impact of different scoring methods (Sensi et al 2000)
- whether dimensions of performance such as knowledge and understanding, skill in application and professional behaviours are assessed (Plasschaert et al 2002)
- ambiguity in description and classification of required performance levels (Dolan 2003, Wang et al 2000)
- the issues of cross institutional consensus on educational objectives and outcome measures (Kurth et al 2001).

Concerns regarding valid and reliable measurement of student competencies when assessing workplace performance has in the past led to medical education emphasising standardised and controlled assessments such as Objective Structured Clinical Examinations (OSCEs) and the use of standardised patients. Other professions, including nursing (Govaerts et al 2002) and physiotherapy, have followed suit. While reliability of assessment will be enhanced by the standardised testing, the validity of such controlled examination procedures has been challenged because, as proposed earlier and highlighted in Chapter 3, competence under controlled conditions may not be an adequate surrogate for performance under the complex and uncertain conditions encountered in usual practice. In addition, important professional attributes such as reflection and willingness to learn and adopt new practices is not easily assessed under controlled conditions.

Norcini (2003a) argues that we should develop and refine performance-based assessments. Ideal assessment procedures should facilitate evaluation of the complex domains of competency in the context of the practice environment within which competence is desirable. Assessment of habitual performance in the clinical environment is essential for making judgements about clinical competence and professional behaviours and, importantly, for guiding students towards expected standards of practice performance (Govaerts 2002). In addition, a more longitudinally or context-based assessment enables the important sociocultural perspective of learning to be addressed as students are able to construct their own learning within the context-specific clinical environment (Sfard 1998).

This rationale provides a catalyst for ongoing research into robust and valid assessment instruments and procedures, and was the driver for establishment of the APP tool presented in this chapter. Table 9.1 provides a summary of methods that have been reported for assessing competency in the health professions. All methods of assessment have intrinsic strengths and weaknesses, and assess different aspects of Miller's hierarchy (1990).

METHOD	DESCRIPTION	INFLUENCES ON LEARNING	REFERENCES
Written examinations *Relationship to Miller's hierarchy—knows and knows how*			
Multiple-choice questions Short answer questions Essays Case presentations	Written examination questions	Encourages thinking and development of writing skills Can measure complex cognitive skills if constructed appropriately	Case & Swanson 2000, Schuwirth et al 2001, 2004, Molenaar et al 2004
Patient management problems (PMPs)	Written patient simulations. Information progressively revealed as students progress through material		McGuire 1995, Miller 1990, Newble et al 2000
Computer assisted simulated encounter (CASE)	Computer based, similar to PMPs. Program responds differentially according to student's responses		Edelstein et al 2000, McGuire 1995
Portfolios	Prepared by student with examples of patients examined and treated, analysis of critical incidents. Fosters reflection on development of competence		Carraccio & Englander 2004, McMullan et al 2003, Pitts et al 2001, 2002
Oral examinations *Relationship to Miller's hierarchy—knows and knows how*			
Viva voce	Oral examination, questions are asked and answered orally although there may be an initial written stimulus. Questions seek to assess student's knowledge and problem solving capability	Improves verbal communication skills and 'reasoning in and about action' Provides educator with immediate feedback on learning Student has access to immediate formative feedback from a credible expert	Wass et al (2001)
Presentations	Student makes a formal presentation, e.g. of a case, to an audience including assessor		
Clinical simulations *Relationship to Miller's hierarchy—shows how*			

Objective Structured Clinical Examinations (OSCEs)	A series of independent timed 'stations' designed to assess specific and predetermined clinical skills. Stations may include specific technical tasks, e.g. reading an X-ray, assessing a standardised patient Assessed using either a checklist or global rating scale A minimum of ten stations spread over 3–4 hours thought necessary to achieve sufficiently reliable evidence of student ability (0.85–0.90)	Improves communication skills and 'reasoning in and about action' Encourages thinking and development of specific skills Can measure complex cognitive skills if constructed appropriately Can be tailored to specific learning objectives Student has access to immediate formative feedback	Boulet et al 2003, Manogue et al 2000, Ward & Willis 2006
Standardised patients	Students perform an interview and/or physical examination of an actor trained to portray the same patient on repeated occasions May be incorporated into OSCEs as an individual station. Assessed using checklist or global rating scale		Barrows 1993, Epstein & Hundert 2002, Hampl et al 1999, Tamblyn 1998, Resnick et al 1993
Hi-technology simulations	Simulations involving sophisticated mannequins and computer produced graphics		
Chart stimulated recall	Examiner discusses management of a patient based on patient's chart information (actual or simulated patient and/or chart)		McGuire 1995
Performance–workplace assessments by patients and/or peers *Relationship to Miller's hierarchy—does*			
Patient assessments of student performance	Ratings from patients or clients regarding aspects of care they have received	Promotes understanding of patient perspective and may improve collaborative (patient-centred) practice Emphasises use of skill and knowledge in relevant problem context Student has access to immediate formative feedback from a credible, highly relevant stakeholder	Ilott & Murphy 1997, Norman et al 2002, Violato et al 1997

METHOD	DESCRIPTION	INFLUENCES ON LEARNING	REFERENCES
Peer assessment 360 review process (includes peers, staff and patients) Multi-source feedback	Students assessed (formatively) and/or rated on aspects of clinical competency by peers. Trainees choose at least ten assessors who complete an assessment form (e.g. Team Assessment of Behaviour) privately, sign and return. Assessors chosen should represent a diverse range of professional colleagues, healthcare team members and administrative staff who know the trainee well enough to comment Usually used to assess trainee's professional behaviours	Emphasises use of skill and knowledge in relevant problem context Student has access to feedback from a group of highly relevant stakeholders	Norcini 2003b, Lipner et al 2002 Evans et al 2004, Whitehouse et al 2005
Performance–workplace assessments by supervising clinicians *Relationship to Miller's hierarchy—does*			
Physiotherapy • Clinical Performance Instrument (CPI) • Clinical Internship Evaluation Tool (CIET) • Assessment of Physiotherapy Practice (APP) • Common Assessment Form (CAF) **Speech pathology** • COMPASS™ **Occupational Therapy** • Student Placement Evaluation Form (SPEF) **Medicine** • Mini Clinical Evaluation Exercise (Mini-CEX) • Direct Observation of Procedural Skills (DOPS)	Student is observed working with multiple patients over an extended period of time (4–12 weeks). Formative feedback provided during the clinical unit and summative assessment based on longitudinal evaluation provided at end of the unit. Students assessed on all aspects of clinical competency as described by professional accrediting authorities. Grading of student's overall performance across the unit is performed by a supervising clinician and/or university academic Student observed working with patient and assessed by supervising clinician on aspects of their care. Assessments usually limited to a specific aspect of patient examination or management and take approximately 20 min. Feedback on performance is provided immediately. Students obtain multiple examinations across clinical unit, e.g. six over a 10-week clinical rotation	Promotes authentic context specific learning: • foundation knowledge of health sciences • clinical skills • habits of reflection • professional behaviour • interpersonal skills • integration of relevant and current knowledge into practice Student has access to immediate formative feedback from a credible expert	Allison & Turpin 2004, Dalton et al 2008, Fitzgerald et al 2007, McAllister 2005, Roach et al 2002, Coote et al 2007 Adams 2003, Dolan 2003, Norman 2002, Norcini et al 1995, Wass et al 2001, Ram et al 1999

Table 9.1 Methods used to assess competency of students of the healthcare professions

Maximising assessment that improves performance

It is often assumed that providing ongoing feedback as a form of formative assessment is both natural and easy, but student feedback and previous literature indicates that it is frequently done quite poorly (Ende et al 1995, Hewson & Little 1998). To provide consistently useful assessment and feedback, educators need to monitor their attitudes and biases, the way they design targets for student skill development, and the way they utilise language. Assessment and feedback about assessment can be confounded by educator feelings such as negativity, anxiety, frustration, lack of confidence in their own skills in some areas, or even positive regard for the student. Educators are likely to benefit from opportunities and strategies to use to reflect on the way they assess students. For example, the SMART model proposes that assessment should be delivered using methods that are Specific, Measurable, Achievable, Realistic and Timely (Drucker 1954). These attributes require educators to reflect on how to provide feedback that describes desirable behaviour.

Borrell-Carrió and Epstein (2004) articulate a range of factors that might reduce the quality of clinical decisions and professional performance. These might also be considered as factors that impact on assessment in the clinical environment. Clinical educators are particularly vulnerable to effects of fatigue and of feeling overwhelmed by workload, factors that might translate into an urgency to finish a task or a lack of motivation to model the highest possible standards. Added to this, patient needs and behaviours can complicate the interaction between clinician and student if the clinician feels intimidated or annoyed by patient or student anxiety or hostility.

Educators might be vulnerable to retreating behind what Borrell-Carrió and Epstein (2004) describe as 'low-level decision rules'. These are positions that are taken without reflective evaluation of needs and goals specific to the situation. Some examples are provided in Table 9.2 to illustrate the point and provide non-prescriptive examples of possible alternative (high-level) decisions.

Recognising challenges and bias in the assessment of students

Formative assessment that mimics summative assessment provides the educator with important opportunities to reflect on their own biases that might work for or against the student. If educators recognise there are circumstances such as fatigue or overload that render them vulnerable to retreating behind low-level decisions and responses, they are in a position to introduce habits that facilitate high-level decisions. Borrell-Carrió and Epstein (2004) suggest strategies for minimising practice errors that might be considered in this context. Educators might reflect on when they are at risk of cognitive distortion, prematurely closing on a teaching encounter that warrants additional attention or the use of 'low-level decision rules' and detecting moments when it is necessary to 'reframe the interaction'. As part of basic training in clinical education, a teacher might develop some habitualised cognitive, emotional, and behavioural skills, such as methods to detect states of low cognition and emotional overload, that could lead to dismissing rather than attending to needs of students. Educators could be assisted to cultivate an awareness of states of fatigue and the potential for such fatigue to limit capacity for high-level decisions. They could learn the skill of stepping back from a situation when interaction with the student has ceased to be productive or their ability to provide quality assessment is poor. Leaving a non-productive interaction can enable the opportunity to revisit the interaction at a time when re-engagement or a new perspective is possible. Practical strategies include slowing down,

LOW-LEVEL DECISIONS	HIGH-LEVEL DECISIONS AND REFLECTIVE HABITS
As soon as I met him I knew he was lazy	This student needs strategies to develop attention to desirable performance indicators
She is a good student and can be left to manage patients on her own	This student requires high-level challenges to maintain her motivation and promote development
She is very defensive when I give feedback and does not listen to me	I will write down what you have said and reflect on it and we can discuss this again tomorrow
She really shouldn't be here. She doesn't have enough theoretical knowledge	Why not take some time to re-familiarise yourself with the following learning objectives and we will repeat this challenge tomorrow
He is not acting professionally	For this student I need to explicitly define areas of professional development that require attention and clearly communicate my expectation about the way in which they need to improve
I got quite angry with the student because they had not adequately prepared for the situation	What interfered with my ability to observe, be attentive, or be respectful with this student? What would a trusted peer say about the way I managed this situation?
I don't have time to go over this again, I have a lot of patients to see	How could I be more present with and available to this student?
He is much better than she is	Were there any points at which I felt judgemental about the student in a positive or negative way?
He is not improving, no matter how much help I give him	If there were relevant data that I ignored, what might they be?

Table 9.2 Applying high- and low-level decision rules (Borrell-Carrió & Epstein 2004) to evaluation of student needs

recommending the interaction is deferred to a period following rest or reflection, discussing options with more experienced colleagues, placing a pause into an interaction to enable learning a new pattern of response, and reflecting on the goal of the education process rather than the detail of a specific interaction (Borrell-Carrió & Epstein 2004). In addition to workplace pressures that might induce less than ideal conditions at the educator–student interface, both student and educator are vulnerable to a number of well-documented biases that can affect formative assessment. If an educator allows a global bias about a student (either negative 'devil effect' or positive 'halo effect') to operate beneath interactions, it may be difficult to accurately assess, reward or guide development of performance.

A devil effect would occur if an educator had negative views about an undesirable trait in a student, and this influenced their approach to subsequent interactions and assessments. A simple example would be if a student did not make eye contact and said little during discussions. The educator may assume indifference on the student's part, and judge performance more harshly than they would if they perceived the student as friendly and engaged. The devil effect can also operate to create an impression the student may not be able to rectify. To illustrate with a simple example, at their first clinic the student arrived five minutes late several times in the first week. The educator discusses expectations of punctuality and the student, recognising a need for adjustment in less than rigorous habits, subsequently arrives five minutes early every day for the remainder of the clinic. If the student received a summative report that included a drop in grades associated with punctuality, they would have reason to be unhappy. Anecdotally, students make frequent complaints that these 'sustained judgements' are commonplace.

A devil effect can tarnish educator perspective and lead to inaccurate assumptions. Gilbert & Malone (1995) refer to this as assumption bias about student motivation or ability that can be difficult for the student to counter. A reflective educator might use tricks such as those proposed by Borrell-Carrió and Epstein (2004) to limit the potential for bias to thread its way across repeated assessments.

Critical appraisal of the situation can fill the gap between stereotypical responses that are, on the one hand, the result of our prior experiences and, on the other, reflective, high-order decisions and behaviours. However, even reflective decisions may be prone to biases. In the clinical education context, easily accessible de-biasing techniques are needed. Strategies to ensure attention is paid to the detail of what a student is demonstrating, include structured methods for assessing a performance of a skill based on explicit descriptions of desirable performance, pausing to reflect and asking oneself to take a somewhat remote view of the situation, 'What would a close and respected colleague think about my assessment of this performance?'. These strategies may serve to disentangle a dominant effect of bias and reset attention to observed performance.

A similar effect can occur if the educator has developed a very positive view of a student based on limited exposure to their skills and a 'halo' caused by an unrelated attribute of the student. Care must be taken not to deny the student appropriate guidance, and again self-reflective questioning might mitigate the potential for bias to distort perceptions. Anchoring is a bias that occurs when the mind, in search of a value, seizes upon a random reference point. In clinical education, anchoring bias could occur if two students were concurrently supervised by the same educator and the skills of one are compared to the skills of another, rather than to the target skills that are the requirements of professional accreditation to practice. Confirmation bias is the tendency to seek to confirm, rather than contradict, a prevailing hypothesis and operates to sustain 'halo' and 'devil' effects. Belief perseverance refers to adherence to a theory when the evidence for the theory is disproved. In addition, the desire to avoid cognitive dissonance can cause people to adjust perception so that information that contradicts an established position is ignored. Where these biases operate, in isolation or combination, it may become very difficult for a student to improve their assessment outcomes despite relevant improvements in performance.

Outcome bias may be another important source of bias for assessors to consider. This bias influences people to judge a decision more harshly if they are aware of a bad outcome than they would judge the same decision if they are unaware of the bad outcome (Henriksen & Kaplan 2003). In clinical education, a student whose decision or performance results in patient complications (or improvements) is likely to be assessed more harshly (or favourably) than if there were no observable consequences arising from those actions. Judging single decisions on the basis of their outcomes is problematic because the student has not had a chance to demonstrate learning or reflection arising from knowledge of the outcome. It is also inaccurate because it uses information that was not available at the time the decision was made. Assessing the quality of decisions should be confined to assessment of the way the student approached the problem and its solution.

Reflecting on sources of cognitive bias, and where they might operate in a person's life, is an important step in controlling the dominance that these biases can have over perceptions. A change in stimulus intensity might change educator responses from enjoyment to displeasure, or from cooperative to competitive emotions. A student repeatedly asking the same question or requesting help for the same skill development might change an educator's reaction from interest to irritation. Educators will naturally seek a cognitive alibi for their behaviour and may categorise the student to explain their irritation: 'She has a very irritating manner with the patient', or 'He is a very slow learner'. This type of categorisation might enable premature closure on evaluation of the educational opportunities in a situation, and stifle the relationship required for fruitful modelling of high-level decision making and professional behaviour. It is at this point that the advantage of a reflective approach to the role and responsibilities of the educator and student might enable more thoughtful and productive responses to the student, and assist with developing suitable strategies to deal with apparent difficulties.

Best practice in performance-based assessments in health settings

Epstein (2007) argues that competence is not an endpoint but the habit of performing to a standard that will evolve as systems of care change. On this basis, whatever method is employed to assess competence or performance, it should provide insight into actual performance (what the student does habitually when not observed) as well as the capacity to adapt to change, find, apply and generate new knowledge and demonstrate understanding of health service systems. Assessors are likely to benefit from structured education in the assessment practices and procedures (Page 2004) and should be engaged in the process of refining assessment procedures through feedback and forward planning (Wilson & Scalise 2006), and from a financial cost perspective.

Box 9.2 lists a range of strategies that might be considered to create a positive learning and assessment environment.

BOX 9.2 Strategies for a positive learning and assessment environment

- Outline goals of the assessment
- Create a suitable hierarchy of skill development challenges
- Consider a range of assessment methods including direct observation of performance and a mixture of assessment approaches
- Include assessment (formative or summative) that recognises and rewards skill acquisition
- Be very clear about target behaviours
- Describe targets using the language of measurable behaviours
- Maintain challenge and reward by setting and assessing increasingly challenging targets
- Balance the challenges and variety to maximise enthusiasm and minimise fatigue, e.g. mix patient contact with reflective activities and study away from the patient
- Minimise expressions of frustration, irritation or blame and demonstrate a willingness to explore strategies to advance student skills
- Use reflective practice to evolve and refine positive teacher attitudes
- Model professional skills including reflective practice
- Model high-level decision making with patients and with students
- Recognise emotions or states that mitigate against a positive interaction with the student and revisit the interaction when a more productive encounter is likely
- Develop strategies to reflect on the way that bias might affect educator attitude to a student
- Implement opportunities for clinical educators to develop skills in formative and summative assessment
- Implement ongoing review and refinement of the assessment system.

Developing instruments to measure performance in the clinical context

Since assessment outcomes have 'high stakes' for students (Epstein 2007) and for the quality of the profession, assessment processes should be developed systematically, rigorously tested for quality, and be approved by national bodies or boards of the profession. Consensus about what constitutes entry-level practice standards and clearly defined performance indicators promote profession-wide dialogue regarding the perceived validity of assessment methods, and provide a springboard for evolution and improvement over time.

Underpinning advice regarding the development of high-quality assessment procedures is an assumption that validity is conferred when key learning objectives are clearly defined and agreed upon by clinical educators (Page 2004, Roberts et al 2006, Wilson & Scalise 2006). Matching the range of assessment targets to a suitable range of assessment procedures, known as blueprinting, supports this process (Roberts et al 2006). Sometimes objectives are 'set' by accreditation bodies but invariably there are details in the assessment process that must be resolved through a consensus process with educators (van der Vleuten 1996).

Reliability

Reliability of clinical assessment refers to the extent to which assessment of competency yields relatively consistent outcomes. It is typically approached through evaluation of agreement across educators on assessment scores. There will always be some disagreement, and defining the limits of tolerable disagreement is challenging. At the very least, agreement regarding what constitutes adequate competency should be established with a degree of precision that correlates with the consequences of error. When there would be serious consequences associated with awarding qualification in the absence of competency, the potential for error should be studied exhaustively.

When examination conditions can be standardised (e.g. using OSCEs) variability in the conditions of examination can be controlled, limiting the influence that these variations might play in the outcomes of assessment. When assessment of performance takes place at the health delivery interface, many factors combine to influence student performance and subsequent assessment outcomes. Some of these have already been discussed. They include patient, student and educator emotional states and behaviours, the complexities of individual patient circumstances and health needs, and students' past experience with the level of challenge confronted under assessment procedures. These conditions are likely to decrease the reliability of one-off assessments.

Conversely, a student assessed longitudinally across a range of circumstances and by a number of assessors has repeated opportunities to demonstrate both ability and growth in ability. In these conditions, assessment outcomes might intuitively be considered to more reliably reflect true ability, as the averaging of repeated measurements typically narrows error bands for measurements taken under highly controlled experimental conditions. However determining reliability of assessments under circumstances when student ability is expected to change presents an added challenge. With adequate funding, student performance could be concurrently monitored and assessed by more than one educator, and assessment procedures refined until adequate concordance in grading is achieved. However even if acceptable error is identified under such an approach, it is likely that, occasionally, unacceptable variation in assessment will still occur across individual assessors. A pragmatic and perhaps less costly approach to optimising reliability is to implement effective education in best practice in student assessment and strategies for developing a shared vision of expectations of performance. If this results in graduates who are typically considered competent, the profession might infer that assessment procedures had adequate reliability.

Validity

There are many approaches to establishing instrument validity. Some consider the assessment procedures and ask whether, on the face of it, they appear to measure the underlying construct of interest (in this case, competence in the clinical context). Others compare scores obtained using defined assessment procedures to other evidence of student ability (clinical assessment scores might be compared to OSCE grades or paper-based problem-solving skills). Other methods involve studying the consistency of item difficulty across different students, assuming that if items are measuring a single underlying construct and item difficulty is consistent across students, that higher performing students will have more of the underlying construct; that is, be more competent. The Standards for Educational and Psychological Testing (American Educational Research Association 1999) take the approach that validity is not an inherent quality of a test but rather that evidence for the validity of a particular application of a test must be established. The standards categorise evidence for test validity based on content, response processes, internal structure, relations to other variables and feedback regarding the consequences of using an instrument.

Validity based on content

It is generally considered important that assessment procedures appear to measure the underlying construct of interest. Items included in the assessment of clinical competence are invariably determined by profession-specific educators. A transparent consensus approach with input from an appropriate spectrum of key stakeholders, such as national accrediting bodies, graduate employers, educators who use the assessment procedures and a broad spectrum of practitioners, typically results in agreement regarding face validity. A study of face validity might also include examination of the way in which items on a test are applied and interpreted by assessors. One approach to this is to conduct 'talk aloud' interviews. In this approach, while conducting a real-time assessment, the assessor explains their reasoning behind scoring of items to an investigator. Concordance across assessors might be interpreted as evidence of face validity.

Validity evidence based on internal structure

Validity can be inferred from a study of the pattern in scores for a cohort. If the assessment procedures are measuring an underlying construct, for example competency, higher scores should indicate greater competency. A variety of statistical approaches are used to examine the internal structure of assessment instruments. Factor analysis, item-item and item-total correlations, Cronbach alpha and Rasch analysis are frequently utilised strategies.

Validity based on relations to other variables

A relatively common approach to assessment of validity is to compare total scores obtained for assessment to measures taken using a simple global rating scale. Students might, for example, be assessed using an instrument with twenty items each ranked from 0 to 5 and a total score out of 100 awarded. These scores can then be compared with outcomes when educators are asked to rank the student as 'fail, pass, good, very good, exceptional'. This enables standard setting (determining the range of scores typically associated with pass levels) and also enables validation against the reference standard. A comprehensive description of an approach to standard setting is reported by Roberts et al (2006). Significantly higher scores should be seen for students in successive global scale categories, and there should be strong correlations between rating categories and assessment scores.

Validity based on feedback from the profession

Another method of validation is feedback from graduate employers. If assessment procedures are valid, employers should be satisfied with pass graduates and their degree of satisfaction with graduate performance should be greater for students with higher assessment scores than for lower assessment scores. This method of validation is important to professions to ensure that graduates arrive work-ready, but also able to demonstrate rapid change and development in their graduate skills in the period immediately following employment. There is no published evidence that performance measured six months after joining the workforce has any relationship to skills gained as an undergraduate.

Instrument development

The ideas presented in this chapter arose from collaboration between Australian physiotherapists to develop a standardised system, the Assessment of Physiotherapy Practice (APP) instrument, for assessing the clinical performance of physiotherapy students.

In 2006 there were thirteen entry-level physiotherapy programs in Australia. For graduates to be eligible for registration to practise as a physiotherapist on graduation, programs must be accredited by the Australian Physiotherapy Council (formerly the Australian Council of Physiotherapy Regulating Authorities). The Australian Standards for Physiotherapy provide the blueprint that all programs follow to ensure all graduates achieve a minimum set of competencies.

Despite this national accreditation process and single set of competency standards, each physiotherapy program had developed its own instrument to assess student competence in the clinical setting. Importantly, the reliability and validity was unknown. This variation in assessment practices reflects the proposal by Newble et al (1994) that educational methods are commonly based on historical practices or a best guess approach by educators. For clinical educators accepting students from multiple programs, the diversity of assessment forms and supporting documentation represented a substantial and unnecessary burden. As new physiotherapy programs commenced, this burden was multiplied. In 2005, with the support of all universities in Australia and New Zealand, a group of researchers led a project to develop a single national assessment tool. The test development was supported by a grant from the Carrick Institute for Learning and Teaching in Higher Education Ltd. The process of instrument development was planned with consideration of:

- feasibility of the instrument for monitoring and measuring performance in the practice environment
- utility of the instrument for educators and students. For educators, the instrument needed to provide a vehicle for valid assessment of performance and for providing suitable formative feedback to guide the development of desirable performance. For students, the instrument needed to provide a vehicle for appropriate reflection and unambiguous development of performance targets

- validity of the measurements
- reliability of assessment outcomes
- refinement of the instrument utilising feedback from educators and students
- alignment of the instrument with best practice in assessment.

The steps in the development of the APP are shown in Figure 9.2.

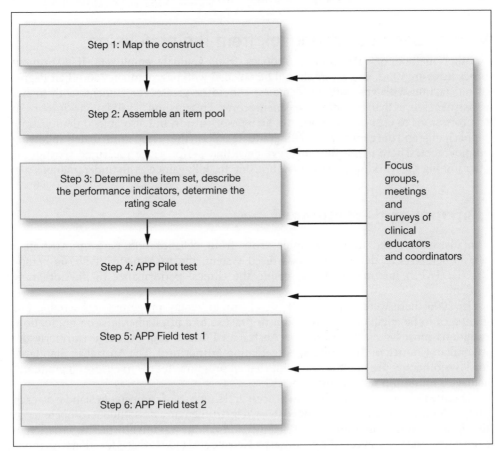

Figure 9.2 Steps in the development of the APP

Step 1   Map the construct

A construct map is a visual tool for clarifying the underlying construct to be measured by the instrument, in this case 'clinical competence'. Clinical competence can be thought of as a continuum of performance from very poor (incompetent) through to very high levels of competence, and individual students may demonstrate more or less of the variable. A construct map for the APP is shown in Figure 9.3.

Construct domains were determined from an exhaustive examination of existing instruments and relevant publications, such as the Australian Standards for Physiotherapy. Eight domains were identified:

1 communication
2 professional behaviour

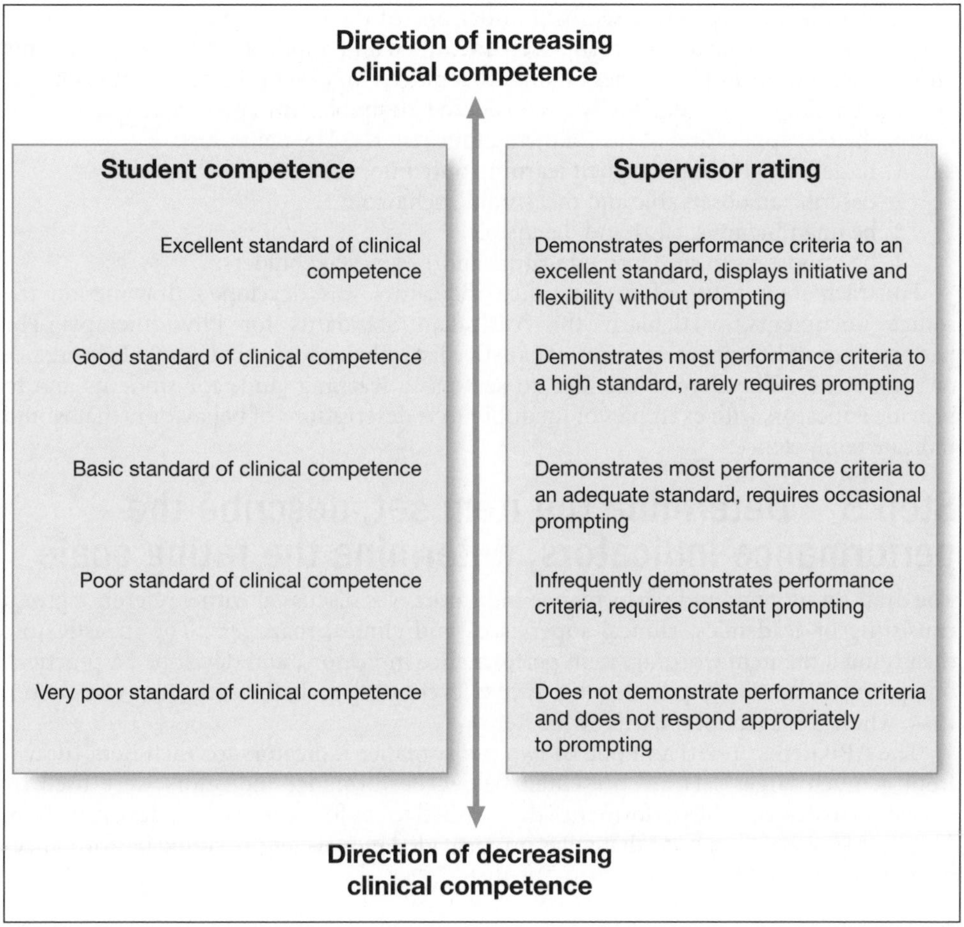

Figure 9.3 Construct map for the APP

3 assessment
4 analysis
5 planning
6 intervention
7 evidence-based practice
8 risk management.

Step 2   Assemble an item pool

An item pool was assembled by drawing items from a broad range of relevant sources:
- all existing instruments in use in Australia and New Zealand
- Australian Physiotherapy competency standards (ACOPRA 2002)
- Australian Standards for Physiotherapy (APC 2006)
- National Patient Safety Framework (Australian Council for Safety and Quality in Health Care 2005)
- National OT competency assessment document (Allison & Turpin 2004)
- The Australian Council on Healthcare Standards, EQuIP Standards (2002).

All identified items were assembled under one of the relevant eight domains. Items in common across source documents were identified and duplicates removed. As a finite and relevant number of assessment items are required for practical assessment of clinical skills, a parsimonious item set was considered desirable. Initial item reduction was approached by application of the following four criteria. The item must:

    1 target one attribute (explicit learning outcome)
    2 describe an observable and measurable behaviour
    3 be unambiguous, clear and defensible
    4 be important to students, educators and/or key stakeholders.

For each item a list of performance indicators was developed drawing on the source documents, particularly the Australian Standards for Physiotherapy. The performance indicators were a non-exhaustive list of behaviours that would be evidence of competence. These were intended to serve as a learning guide for students and to provide educators with examples of unambiguous descriptions of behaviours that would indicate competence.

Step 3   Determine the item set, describe the performance indicators, determine the rating scale

The draft set of items and performance indicators was discussed with a reference group consisting of academics, clinical supervisors and clinical managers. The investigators then refined the item wording, item performance indicators, and developed a practical, one-page test layout for pilot testing. A five-level rating scale for each item was chosen (0–4, where 2 is a pass standard for the item).

The APP items (1–20) and one or two performance indicators for each item (drawn from a much larger set) are presented below. Performance indicators were used by educators to describe the performance they wished to see for improved grades on an item. They were (necessarily) not exhaustive, but provided models for providing performance-based feedback and targets.

PROFESSIONAL BEHAVIOUR

    1 Demonstrates an understanding of patient–client rights and consent
- allows sufficient time to discuss the risks and benefits of the proposed treatment with patient–client and carers
- advises supervisor or other appropriate person if a patient–client might be at risk

    2 Demonstrates commitment to learning
- responds in a positive manner to questions, suggestions and/or constructive feedback

    3 Demonstrates practice that is ethical and in accordance with relevant legal and regulatory requirements
- follows policies and procedures of the facility

    4 Demonstrates teamwork
- contributes appropriately in team meetings

COMMUNICATION

    5 Communicates effectively and appropriately—verbal/non-verbal
- greets others appropriately

    6 Communicates effectively and appropriately—written
- writes legibly

ASSESSMENT

7 Conducts an appropriate patient–client interview (subjective assessment)
   - positions person safely and comfortably for interview
8 Selects appropriate methods for measurement of relevant health indicators
   - chooses appropriate methods and instruments to measure identified outcomes across relevant assessment domains, e.g. impairment, activity limitations, participation restriction, wellbeing and satisfaction with care
9 Performs appropriate assessment procedures (physical assessment)
   - sensibly modifies assessment in response to patient–client profile, feedback and relevant findings

ANALYSIS

10 Appropriately interprets assessment findings
   - describes the implications of test results
11 Identifies and prioritises patient's–client's problems
   - generates a list of problems from the assessment

PLANNING

12 Sets realistic short- and long-term goals with the patient–client
   - formulates goals that are specific, measurable, achievable, relevant and timely
13 Collaborates with patient–client to select appropriate intervention
   - engages with patient–client to explain assessment findings, discuss intervention strategies and develop an acceptable plan

INTERVENTION

14 Performs interventions appropriately
   - considers the scheduling of treatment in relation to other procedures, e.g. medication for pain, wound care
15 Is an effective educator and health promoter
   - demonstrates skill in patient–client education, e.g. understands the principles of adult learning
   - demonstrates skills in conducting group sessions
16 Monitors the effects of intervention
   - incorporates relevant evaluation procedures within the physiotherapy plan
17 Progresses intervention appropriately
   - modifications, continuation or cessation of intervention are made in consultation with the patient–client, based on best available evidence
18 Undertakes discharge planning
   - begins discharge planning in collaboration with the healthcare team at the time of the initial episode of care

EVIDENCE-BASED PRACTICE

19 Applies evidence-based practice in patient care
   - assists patient–client and carers to identify reliable and accurate health information

RISK MANAGEMENT

20 Identifies adverse events and near misses, and minimises risk associated with assessment and interventions
   - complies with workplace guidelines on patient–client handling

Step 4   Pilot test

Data were collected across one semester from students at one university undertaking either their first major clinical placement in third year or the final two placements in fourth year. Analysis of the pilot data indicated the data had adequate fit to the chosen measurement model (Rasch Partial Credit Model), the rating scale was operating as intended, the items were sufficiently targeting the intended performance, and the instrument could discriminate at least four levels of competence. Feedback from clinical educators using the new assessment form was generally positive and was used to refine the instrument.

Steps 5 and 6   Field tests

The APP was used either as the primary assessment instrument or administered in parallel with an existing instrument at a total of nine universities in Australia and New Zealand across two semesters in 2007–08. Analysis of data from the first field trial resulted in minor changes to wording of some items, the collapsing of the analysis and planning items into a single domain, and modifications to the performance indicators.

Validity evidence based on content

Content validity was derived from the process of development that identified a large item pool from all relevant sources and used a set of decision rules to select the final item set. There is broad agreement by the physiotherapy profession about the competencies required for practice. In focus groups and via feedback from clinical educators there was agreement that items were appropriate.

Validity evidence based on response processes

Clinical educators use the APP to provide both formative and summative assessment of physiotherapy student performance. It was important to explore whether the educators found the APP acceptable, were interpreting the items, performance indicators and response scale as intended, and to identify any aspects of the instrument that were ambiguous or inconsistently interpreted. These response processes were examined by surveys, focus groups and 'talk aloud' interviews with clinical educators.

Validity evidence based on internal structure

Evidence from internal structures was sought using Rasch analysis to examine the extent to which observed patterns of responses fit the pattern expected by the model. Person ability and item difficulty were calibrated onto a common interval scale (logits). Analysis examined the functioning of the rating scale, overall fit of data to the model, the fit of individual items and persons to the model, and the stability of item functioning based on variables other than student performance (e.g. by gender or type of placement).

On each item, students were rated on a five-level response scale from poor to excellent demonstration of competence. The expectation is that as student ability increases, the probability they would be rated at a higher level would increase in an ordered fashion from low to high performance. Analysis of the APP data showed that educators were using the five-level response scale as intended. Figure 9.4 shows the category probability curve for the item 'Demonstrates an understanding of patient–client rights and consent'.

Student performance on the logit scale (horizontal axis) ranges from less competent on the left (negative values) to more competent on the right. The five levels of the rating scale have a regular pattern showing that each response option becomes the more

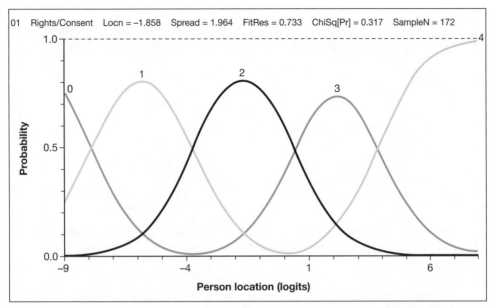

01   Rights/Consent   Locn = −1.858   Spread = 1.964   FitRes = 0.733   ChiSq[Pr] = 0.317   SampleN = 172

Figure 9.4 The category probability curve for the item 'Demonstrates an understanding of patient–client rights and consent'

probable rating as student competence increases. The 'threshold' between each response is the point at which two adjacent responses become equally probable.

Figure 9.5 shows the sequence or hierarchy of difficulty of the twenty competencies on the APP. This allows students and educators to see which clinical competencies are easier to acquire, such as communication and professional behaviours, and those that are more difficult and therefore can be expected to take longer, for example evidence-based practice, analysis and planning.

Reliability

The Person Separation Index (PSI) provides an indication of how many strata of ability a test can discriminate amongst (Wright & Masters 1982). The PSI is a reliability coefficient and for the APP the PSI is >0.9, indicating the test can discriminate four or more levels of competence.

Applying the APP

The APP is currently utilised for both formative and summative assessment, fulfilling the requirement of guiding behaviours expected during summative assessment, discussed earlier in this chapter. Each item is scored against the behaviour expected of a 'day one' new graduate. Clinical educators are asked to advise students regarding behaviours they wish to see in order to award a higher score for each item. Students are asked to request information from educators about behaviours they need to demonstrate in order to achieve higher item scores. Some universities are using cumulative longitudinal evaluation of practice performance to award an 'end of placement' grade, while others are applying 'exit examinations' in addition to cumulative assessment processes. Standard setting is

First clinical placement: easiest to hardest (av. location)		Final clinical placement: easiest to hardest (av. location)	
1	Client rights–consent	3	Ethical practice
2	Commitment to learning	2	Commitment to learning
4	Teamwork	1	Client rights–consent
3	Ethical practice	6	Communication—written
8	Selects outcome measures	4	Teamwork
6	Communication—written	7	Patient interview
17	Progresses intervention	14	Performs interventions
11	Identifies/prioritises problems	20	Minimises risk
16	Monitors effect of intervention	19	Applies EBP
5	Communication—verbal/non-verbal	5	Communication—verbal/non-verbal
15	Effective educator	13	Selects appropriate intervention
20	Minimises risk	18	Discharge planning
13	Selects appropriate intervention	12	Sets realistic short- and long-term goals
12	Sets realistic short- and long-term goals	16	Monitors effect of intervention
7	Patient interview	9	Physical examination
14	Performs interventions	8	Selects outcome measures
9	Physical examination	17	Progresses intervention
19	Applies EBP	10	Interprets assessment findings
18	Discharge planning	11	Identifies/prioritises problems
10	Interprets assessment findings	15	Effective educator

Figure 9.5 APP item average location showing hierarchy of difficulty of the twenty competencies. Numbers represent the APP item

an option particularly during early experiences in practice where students are forming the expectations of their performance.

An advantage of marking students against graduate standards is that, theoretically at least, all assessors are assessing against the same standard. The results from focus group discussions about entry level and beginning physiotherapist standards has demonstrated a clear consensus from clinical educators regarding a global definition of minimally competent performance. The alternative model of grading students against 'the expected competency during the first practice block in third year' or 'the expected competency during the last practice block in fourth year' reduces confidence that consensus in scale use is operating. The target of clinical education is acquisition of a minimum acceptable level of skills, and this target enables ranking of students relative to a common standard.

A disadvantage is that invariably high performing students are disappointed with lower grades that are predictable during their first exposure to a practice interface. Universities have taken the option to make grade adjustments that acknowledge exemplary performers within the mixture of obtained grades. A difficulty that has been encountered is achieving unanimous consensus regarding specific grades awarded to a (pre-recorded) performance of a task, but from one perspective this might be considered an advantage of the instrument. Differences in views regarding specific desirable attributes and item grades have previously been obscured by the individualised rating systems applied across universities. A common standard has enabled discussion regarding the quality of specific performance and how it can be recognised. Teaching DVDs have been developed to enable groups of educators to share views on ratings of standardised performances and, as these are refined with feedback, greater consensus is anticipated. Sources of systematic differences between those making the ratings will be identified across time, and specific training to deal with these anticipated differences can be built into support material.

Applicability of this model to wider clinical education settings

Many of the items on the APP are drawn down from generic competencies expected of all healthcare providers. Therefore application of these instrument development steps and modification of the APP to suit the needs and profession-specific standards of other professions presents as an option. Changing the performance indicators and retaining items would enable significant translation across disciplines.

The APP was developed and applied within the constraints of a dynamic and unpredictable clinical environment. This is a key strength of the measuring tool and ensures that it is reliable, at the same time as being responsive to sociocultural factors in the clinical education environment. It has been challenging to consider how APP reliability (other than the reliability described by the PSI) might be assessed in this context. Even if two of the people doing the ratings, watching the same performance, graded a student in an acceptably similar way, we would have no assurances that every educator in every situation would demonstrate comparable reliability. Comfort in this uncertainty arises from longitudinal monitoring to inform assessment (the student is supervised in a large number of clinical interactions) and typically assessed by more than one educator. Underpinning this comfort is a hope that averages will smooth random minor irregularities and extreme outcomes will be overshadowed by central tendencies in most scores.

The APP has been designed to assist both students and educators. In enabling structured formative feedback, it compels discussion that provides both parties with the opportunity to design a path to achieve specific desirable skills. In particular, it assists both parties to articulate and understand the skills required in clinical learning. Skills in domains, rather than specific performances, are graded, and the comprehensive categories allow structured feedback on the range of circumstances that confront students, educators and patients. The importance of empowering the student to ask for explicit direction and encouraging educators to provide explicit guidance facilitates a two-way dialogue about shared goals, provides students with clear direction, and works against the potential for educator bias.

References

ACOPRA (Australian Council of Physiotherapy Regulating Authorities) 2002 Standards for accreditation of physiotherapy programs at the level of higher education awards

Adams EJ 2003 Best practices in clinical assessment. Health Sciences, University of Sydney

Allison H, Turpin MJ 2004 Development of the student placement evaluation form: a tool for assessing student fieldwork performance. Australian Journal of Occupational Therapy Sep 51(3):125–132

American Educational Research Association, American Psychological Association, National Council on Measurement in Education 1999 Standards for educational and psychological testing. Washington, American Educational Research Association

Australian Council for Safety and Quality in Health Care 2005 National patient safety education framework. Commonwealth of Australia, Canberra

Australian Council on Healthcare Standards (ACHS) 2002 EQuIP Standards, 3rd edn. ACHS

Australian Physiotherapy Council (APC) 2006 Australian standards for physiotherapy. APC, Canberra

Barrows HS 1993 An overview of the uses of standardised patients for teaching and evaluating clinical skills: AAMC. Academic Medicine 68:443–451

Borrell-Carrió F, Epstein R 2004 Preventing errors in clinical practice: a call for self-awareness. Annals of Family Medicine 2:310–316

Boud D 1995 Assessment and learning: contradictory or complementary? In: Knight P (ed) Assessment for learning in higher education. Kogan Page, London, p 35–48

Boulet JR, DeChamplain AF, McKinley DW 2003 Setting defensible performance standards on OSCEs and standardised patient examinations. Medical Teacher 25(3):245–249

Carraccio C, Englander R 2004 Evaluating competence using a portfolio: a literature review and web-based application to the ACGME competencies. Teaching and Learning in Medicine 16:381–387

Case S, Swanson D 2000 Constructing written test questions for the basic and clinical sciences, 3rd edn. National Board of Medical Examiners, Philadelphia

Coote S, Alpine L, Cassidy C, Loughnane M, McMahon S, Meldrum D, O'Connor A, O'Mahoney M 2007 The development and evaluation of a common assessment form for physiotherapy practice education in Ireland. Physiotherapy Ireland 28(2):6–10

Dalton MB, Keating J, Davidson M 2008 The assessment of physiotherapy practice (APP): pilot trial results. The 13th Ottawa International Conference on Clinical Competence, Melbourne, Australia

Dolan 2003 Assessing student nurse clinical competency: will we ever get it right? Journal of Clinical Nursing 12(1):132–141

Drucker PF 1954 The practice of management. Harper & Row, New York

Edelstein RA, Reid HM, Usatine R et al 2000 A comparative study of measures to evaluate medical students performances. Academic Medicine 75(8):825–833

Ende J, Pomerantz A, Erickson F 1995 Preceptors' strategies for correcting residents in an ambulatory care medicine setting: a qualitative analysis. Academic Medicine 70:224–229

Epstein RM 2007 Assessment in medical education. New England Journal of Medicine 356: 387–396

Epstein RM, Hundert EM 2002 Defining and assessing professional competence. Journal of the American Medical Association 287(2):226–235

Evans R, Elwyn G, Edwards A 2004 Review of instruments for peer assessment of physicians. British Medical Journal 328:1240–1243

Fitzgerald LM, Delitto A, Irrgang JJ 2007 Validation of the clinical internship evaluation tool. Physical Therapy 87(7):844–860

Gilbert DT, Malone PS 1995 The correspondence bias. Psychological Bulletin 117(1):21–38

Govaerts JJB, van der Vleuten C, Schuwirth LWT 2002 Optimising the reproducibility of a performance-based test in midwifery education. Advances in Health Sciences Education 7:133–145

Hampl J, Herbold NH, Schneider MA et al 1999 Using standardized patients to train and evaluate dietetics students. Journal of the American Dietetic Association 99(9):1094–1098

Harden RM, Gleeson FA 1979 Assessment of clinical competence using an objective structured clinical examination (OSCE). Medical Education 13:41–54

Henriksen K, Kaplan H 2003 Hindsight bias, outcome knowledge and adaptive learning. Quality and Safety in Health Care 12(suppl 2):ii46–ii50

Hewson M, Little M 1998 Giving feedback in medical education. Journal of General Internal Medicine 13:111–117

Ilott I, Murphy R 1997 Feelings and failing in professional training: the assessor's dilemma. Assessment and Evaluation in Higher Education, 22(3):307–316

Kurth RJ, Irigoyen MM, Schmidt HJ 2001 Structuring student learning in the primary care setting: Where is the evidence? Journal of Evaluation in Clinical Practice 7(3):325–333

Lave J, Wenger E 1991 Situated learning: legitimate peripheral participation. Cambridge University Press, UK

Lipner RS, Blank LL, Leas BF, Fortna GS 2002 The value of patient and peer ratings in recertification. Academic Medicine 77(suppl 10):S64–S66

McAllister S 2005 Competency based assessment of speech pathology students' performance in the workplace. PhD thesis, University of Sydney, Sydney

McGuire CH 1995 Reflections of a maverick measurement maven. Journal of the American Medical Association 274(9):735–740

McMullen M, Endacott R, Gray MA 2003 Portfolios and assessment of competence: a review of the literature. Journal of Advanced Nursing 41(3):283–294

Manogue M, Kelly M, Masaryk SB 2000 Evolving methods of assessment. European Journal of Dental Education 6(3):53–66

Masters GN 1999 Measuring performance: The challenge of assessment. Independent Education 29(1):18–21

Miller GE 1990 The assessment of clinical skills/competence/performance. Academic Medicine 65S:63–67

Molenaar WM, Reinders JJ, Koopmans SA 2004 Written case reports as assessment of the elective student clerkship: consistency of central grading and comparison with ratings of clinical performance. Medical Teacher 26(4):301–304

Molloy EK 2006 Insights into the formal feedback culture in physiotherapy clinical education. School of Physiotherapy, and Department of Education, University of Melbourne, Melbourne

National Patient Safety Education Framework 2005 Australian Council for Safety and Quality. Online. Available: http://www.patientsafety.org.au/pdfdocs/national_patient_safety_education_framework.pdf Accessed 9 Jan 2009

Newble D, Jolly B, Wakeford R 1994 The certification and recertification of doctors: issues in the assessment of clinical competence. Cambridge University Press, UK

Newble D, Norman G, van der Vleuten C 2000 Assessing clinical reasoning. In: Higgs J, Jones M (eds) Clinical reasoning in the health professions, 2nd edn. Butterworth-Heinemann, Oxford, p 9156–9165

Norcini JJ 2003a ABC of learning and teaching in medicine: work-based assessment. British Medical Journal 326(7392):753–755

Norcini JJ 2003b Peer assessment of competence. Medical Education 37:539–543

Norcini JJ, Blank L, Arnold GK, Kimball HR 1995 The Mini-CEX (clinical evaluation exercise): a preliminary investigation. Annals of Internal Medicine 123:795–799

Norman IJ, Watson R, Murrells T 2002 The validity and reliability of methods to assess the competence to practise of pre-registration nursing and midwifery students. International Journal of Nursing Studies, 39:133–145

Oldmeadow L 1996 Developing clinical competence: a mastery pathway. Australian Journal of Physiotherapy 42(1):37–44

Page G 2004 Assessment of fitness to practise. Paper presented at the Australian and New Zealand Association of Medical Education Annual Conference 2004, Adelaide, South Australia

Petrusa A 2002 Clinical performance assessments. In: Norman G, van der Vleuten CPM, Newble DI (eds) International handbook of research in medical education. Kluwer Academic, London, p 673–709

Pitts J, Coles C, Thomas P 2001 Enhancing reliability in portfolio assessment: 'Shaping' the portfolio. Medical Teacher 23(4):351–356

Pitts J, Coles C, Thomas P 2002 Enhancing reliability in portfolio assessment: discussions between assessors. Medical Teacher 24(2):197–201

Plasschaert A, Boyd M, Andrieu S et al 2002 Development of professional competencies. European Journal of Dental Education 6(3):33–44

Ram P, Grol R, Rethans JJ, Schouten B, van der Vleuten CPM, Kester A 1999 Assessment of general practitioners by video observation of communicative and medical performance in daily practice: issues of validity, reliability and feasibility. Medical Education 33:447–454

Resnick RK, Blackmore D, Cohen R et al 1993 An objective structured clinical examination for the licentiate of the medical council of Canada: from research to reality. Academic Medicine 68:suppl:S4–S6

Rethans JJ, Norcini JJ, Baron-Maldonado M et al 2002 The relationship between competence and performance: implications for assessing practice performance. Medical Education 36(10):901–909

Roach K, Gandy J, Deusinger S et al 2002 The development and testing of APTA clinical performance instruments. Physical Therapy 82(4):329–353

Roberts C, Newble D, Jolly B et al 2006 Assuring the quality of high-stakes undergraduate assessments of clinical competence. Medical Teacher 28(6):535–543

Schuwirth LW, Verheggen MM, van der Vleuten CP et al 2001 Do short cases elicit different thinking processes than factual knowledge questions do? Medical Education 35:348–356

Schuwirth LW, van der Vleuten CP 2004 Different written assessment methods: what can be said about their strengths and weaknesses? Medical Education 38:974–979

Sensi S, Pace-Palitti V, Merlitti D et al 2000 Impact of different scoring methods on the clinical skills assessment of internal medicine students. Medical Teacher 22(6):601–603

Sfard A 1998 On two metaphors for learning and the dangers of choosing just one. Educational Researcher 27(2):4–13

Struber J 2004 What future physiotherapy? walking together—side by side. Queensland Health Conference, Queensland Health

Tamblyn RM 1998 Use of standardised patients in the assessment of medical practice. Canadian Medical Association Journal 158:205–207

van der Vleuten CPM 1996 The assessment of professional competence: developments, research and practical implications. Advanced Health Science Education 1:41–67

van der Vleuten CPM 2000 Validity of final examinations in undergraduate medical training. British Medical Journal 321:1217–1219

Violato C, Marini A, Toews J et al 1997 Feasibility and psychometric properties of using peers, consulting physicians, co-workers, and patient to assess physicians. Academic Medicine 72:suppl 1:S82–S84

Wang T, Kolen MJ, Harris DJ 2000 Psychometric properties of scale scores and performance levels for performance assessments using polytomous IRT. Journal of Educational Measurement 37(2):141–162

Ward H, Willis A 2006 Assessing advanced clinical practice skills: Helen Ward and Annaliese Willis show how the development of an objective structured clinical assessment (OSCA) has enabled assessment of nurse practitioner advanced practice clinical skills at Masters level. Primary Health Care 16(3):22–24

Wass V, van der Vleuten C, Shatzer J, Jones R 2001 Assessment of clinical competence. Lancet 357(9260):945–949

Wiggins G 1989 A true test: toward more authentic and equitable assessment. Phi Delta Kappan 71(9):703–713

Whitehouse AB, Hassell A, Wood L, Wall D, Walzman M, Campbell I 2005 Development and reliability testing of TAB, a new form for 360° assessment of senior house officers' professional behaviour, as specified by the General Medical Council. Medical Teacher 27:252–258

Wilson M, Scalise K 2006 Assessment to improve learning in higher education: the BEAR assessment system. Higher Education 52:635–663

Wright BD, Masters GN 1982 Rating scale analysis. Mesa Press, Chicago

CHAPTER 10

Ethics in clinical education

Clare Delany, Lynn Gillam and Rosalind McDougall

THEORIES

Theories about the nature and source of knowledge in clinical practice are referred to as *practice epistemology*. Methods of teaching practice knowledge is referred to as *educational pedagogy*. In the area of ethics teaching, being clear about the epistemological basis of clinical ethics knowledge provides a means to more carefully match clinical ethics education content and pedagogy with the opportunities and barriers that influence its application in practice.

USING THEORIES TO INFORM EDUCATION PRACTICE AND RESEARCH

When planning ethics curricula for clinical education contexts, it is important to be aware of which strand or epistemological basis is informing the teaching goals and methods. Acting ethically in clinical practice involves being able to critically consider a range of options. It may also require skills in advocacy from a patient or health practitioner level, or from a broader institutional or health policy level. Clinical ethics education requires explication of clear goals and outcomes in required knowledge and skills.

USING THEORIES TO INFORM EDUCATION METHODS

Example: Marie, a 16 year old, has progressive paralysis and been diagnosed with a spinal tumour. She will progress to needing life support. Her parents do not want the doctors, nurses or allied health practitioners to inform her of the cause of her paralysis or the prognosis. They would like Marie to maintain some hope that she will recover and they see no point in telling her of the inevitable prognosis.

Using a case study such as this or asking students for cases they encounter in clinical placements is a common teaching method in ethics education. Each of the strands of ethics education introduced in this chapter might be used to frame ways to approach the ethical issues in this case, and would result in different considerations of appropriate ethical actions. A process of ethical decision making with reference to established ethical principles would focus on which principles were important and how to weigh up their relevance to the case. Focusing on advocacy for the patient or the patient's family would result in a different emphasis on ethical action, as would adopting a particular caring attitude, acting with integrity and acting according to defined and established professional standards. All of these approaches would be relevant to inform the discussion about ethically appropriate actions in this case.

When teaching ethics using case studies or in clinical placements, having a clear understanding of which underlying educational approach is being emphasised provides an important first step. Being clear about the goals of ethics education, their application in clinical cases and, more broadly, in different healthcare workplaces assists students to deal with the range of ethical issues and approaches they will encounter in clinical practice.

Introduction

Ethics education is recognised as an integral component of all health professionals' education. In this chapter, we highlight a number of trends in ethics education for health professionals; trends that can be seen across the different health professions, although some are more prominent in particular health disciplines than others. We refer to these trends as 'strands' in ethics education, because we regard them as representing different aspects or parts of the whole picture of ethics education, rather than as competing interpretations of the whole picture. In identifying these strands, we aim to increase awareness of similarities and differences between themes and issues raised in ethics education in the different health disciplines.

Awareness of a broader range of approaches, and the possibilities for combining them in new ways, suggests ways in which ethics education can be improved to make it more relevant to the needs and experiences of health professionals who practice in a complex, multidisciplinary healthcare environment. We also suggest that within some of the strands lie the beginnings of ideas and resources to address what we argue is the greatest challenge facing ethics education in the health professions, namely the powerful and often very negative influence of the so-called 'hidden curriculum'.

Trends in ethics education in the health professions

Formal ethics education has been occurring in various guises in the curricula of health professional training in many countries since at least the 1970s. There are a variety of approaches to the teaching of ethics, which grow out of different responses to two basic questions on which ethics educators must take a position (whether consciously or not). These questions are: (1) What actually constitutes ethical practice for this profession? and (2) What are the threats to ethical practice? Although there are important differences in the way these questions are answered in medicine, nursing and the various allied health disciplines, it is also notable that some common strands can be identified. Each strand represents a particular understanding of what is important in terms of ethical practice, and what sorts of knowledge, skills and attitudes students need to acquire during their education in order to be ethically competent practitioners.

Viewing ethics education in terms of these strands provides an overview of the key issues and concerns in ethics education, both theoretical and practical. These strands indicate that particular educational issues are not confined to one health discipline but rather cross disciplinary boundaries—a phenomenon which is not so surprising given that professionals from these disciplines often work together in the same institutions, providing care for the same patients.

Strand 1   Ethics as decision making for action

Perhaps the most established and strongest trend in ethics education in the health professions is the focus on ethical decision making. This approach to teaching ethics rests on the assumption that ethical practice is primarily about ethical decision making in the same way as clinical reasoning is seen as vital to clinical practice (Ch 7). In ethics education the aim is to teach students how to reason well, using recognised ethical principles, and hence come to ethically justified decisions. It is assumed that this reasoned ethical decision making is the difficult and central part—having come to a decision the health professional will be able to act to put that decision into practice, and what will flow from this is ethical practice.

In this strand, knowledge of ethical principles and theories is emphasised, as are skills in critical thinking, analysis and decision making. Knowledge of legal and regulatory frameworks is also included. There is little overt attention to ethical attitudes, but there is an implicit focus on the value of rational and dispassionate thought, and on the need for detachment from emotion and personal engagement to take an objective, analytical view. Methods of teaching in this approach typically include didactic instruction about principles and models of decision making. Along with this come case studies aimed at showing how principles and models work in practice, and giving students practice in using knowledge of principles and skills of critical thinking to make their own decisions. Teaching ethical decision making using case studies presumes that students will be willing and able to transfer their skills in ethical analysis to the clinical setting as either students or practitioners.

Seeing ethics education as a matter of teaching ethical decision making is a very strong trend in medical education. In the United Kingdom, the United States and Australia, groups of ethicists and medical educators have put forward a core medical ethics curriculum, articulating the basic content areas necessary to an appropriate undergraduate medical ethics course (Culver et al 1985, Ashcroft et al 1998, ATEAM 2001). A great deal of agreement is evident across these three core curricula with each emphasising ethical theories and concepts as well as various specific issues, such as informed consent, truth telling, end-of-life decisions, research ethics, genetic and reproductive technologies, and resource allocation. These knowledge elements of the curriculum are coupled with the skills of ethical reasoning and, to a lesser extent, communication. Beauchamp and Childress' (2001) framework of four principles governing doctors' relationships with patients—respect for autonomy, beneficence, non-maleficence and justice—has been a particularly influential moral framework in undergraduate medical ethics teaching. The dominance of this framework is evidence for the prevalence among medical ethics educators of the understanding that ethics is about systematic reasoned decision making.

An emphasis on processes of ethical decision-making education is also the standard approach in allied health ethics education (Chapparo & Ranker 2000, Kenny et al 2007, Eaton et al 2003, Barnitt & Partridge 1997). In physiotherapy, for example, ethical reasoning and models of ethical decision making (Purtilo 1999) are considered to be valuable approaches to preparing students for clinical practice, because they share characteristics and features of clinical reasoning. Edwards et al (2005) suggest a number of parallel processes between clinical and ethical reasoning. Both involve deductive reasoning drawing from ethical theories and principles, and both involve recognition of the patients' perspective and surrounding clinical context to inform the reasoning steps (Edwards & Delany 2008).

The approach to ethics education in allied health looks very similar to the framework used by medical practitioners. The knowledge base is virtually identical including, for example, informed consent, respect for patient autonomy and confidentiality. Differences can be found in the emphasis that allied health practitioner literature places on combining the analysis of universal moral theories and biomedical principles with the socially constructed realities and perspectives of patients within particular clinical contexts, but these differences are minor in comparison to the similarities.

In nursing, ethics education is also often understood and presented as primarily a matter of ethical decision making, and can look very similar in style and content to medical and allied health ethics. Knowledge areas given attention include truth-telling, informed consent, confidentiality, end-of-life decision making and allocation of resources, just as they are in medicine and allied health (Fry & Johnstone 2002). Students are taught ethical concepts from moral philosophy, such as autonomy; ethical principles in the Beauchamp and Childress tradition; and are introduced to skills and models for ethical decision making (van Hooft et al 1995, Thompson et al 2000). However nursing differs from the other health disciplines in that this decision-making approach is not universally accepted. Indeed, it is hotly contested and rejected by some, and is certainly not the single predominant approach to teaching nursing ethics. One suggested limitation of a rationally based model of ethical decision making in nursing practice—discussed in Strand 2—is its neglect of the role of emotion and compassion as intrinsic elements of ethical action (Doane et al 2004).

Strand 2   Ethics as character and attitude

A quite different understanding of ethics is to see it primarily in terms of the personal character and attitudes of the health professional, rather than in the decisions they make. This approach to ethics has a long history in the Western philosophical tradition, beginning with Aristotle, and is now commonly referred to as virtue ethics. When virtue ethics is the basis for ethics teaching, teaching methods look very different since they aim at promoting attitudes and character traits, virtues such as honesty, compassion and humility, rather than reasoning skills and conceptual knowledge. In this sort of teaching, methods commonly used are experiential (placing students in particular environments to learn what it feels like, involving students in drama, writing of poetry), and reflection (such as journal or diary keeping). There is generally much less attention given to skills and knowledge in this strand of ethics teaching, although arguably both have a role to play in actually manifesting the relevant virtues or attitudes. In theory, virtue ethics does have a place for both conceptual knowledge and reasoning skills: an agent is supposed to think about what would constitute right action by considering what the virtuous person would do, and by aiming for moderation rather than extremes in the virtues, rather than simply acting on impulse. In practice, this does not receive much attention.

In medicine, this understanding of ethics is secondary to ethics as decision making but is nonetheless still present. Core medical ethics curricula emphasise attitudes such as compassion, honesty and integrity. These are seen as fundamental alongside the content areas and decision-making skills outlined in the previous section. Sophisticated virtue ethics that emphasise character traits of the good doctor has increasingly been a feature of the philosophical literature in medical ethics (Drane 1988, Pellegrino & Thomasma 1993, Oakley & Cocking 2001), and this emphasis on developing the appropriate personal qualities can be particularly substantial in universities where medical ethics education is framed as part of professionalism or packaged as an element of medical humanities.

In allied health, there is often an emphasis on professional attitudes, with students explicitly encouraged to adopt a caring and empathic approach. Here there is a quite tangible, overt rationale. The nature of allied health practice is to engage with, motivate, understand and respond to the patient's individual needs (Poulis 2007, Purtilo 2005, Rogers 2005). Thus, the appropriate attitude is seen as intrinsic to the success of the rehabilitation, acute care and health promotion work of many allied health therapies. Purtilo (2005, p 53) suggests that adopting a caring response as a way of acting ethically means asking 'What does it mean to provide a caring response in this situation?'. Underlying this question is an assumption that caring for a patient, developing a relationship of trust, and making real contact with patients via a caring presence is a valid way of acting ethically. Teaching students to adopt caring dispositions as a means of guiding actions, involves close examination of the meaning of particular attitudes such as empathy and respect (Peloquin 2005). In allied health, attention to caring attitudes generally occurs in combination with an understanding of rigorous and systematic applications of biomedical principles, which are seen as primary components of the teaching of ethics.

In contrast to medicine and allied health, nursing offers a more radical version of this focus on character and attitude in its ethics of care movement. Ethics of care is more radical than virtue ethics because it involves the explicit rejection of abstract principles and reasoning. Ethics of care understands ethical practice solely as a matter of caring: that is, as an orientation of self towards others or a way of being, which has nothing to do with analytical thought. Ethics of care arose partly out of a sense of threat to the ethical practice of nursing from increasing medical technology. Beginning in the 1970s, a number of nursing theorists, including Jean Watson (1979) and Madeleine Leininger (Leininger & McFarland 1995), began to argue that nursing as a profession had become so focused on the technology of healthcare that it had forgotten about caring for the patient as a person. They argued for a philosophy of care which located nursing ethics entirely in the caring relationship between nurse and patient. On this approach, nursing ethics is not at all about decision making, but rather about engaging in a particular type of interpersonal, deeply caring relationship. Nursing curricula which adopt this approach to ethics characteristically see teaching ethics as a matter of moral development, in particular of cultivating and inculcating attitudes of caring, empathy and engagement (Vanlaere & Gastmans 2007), and place emphasis on the experiential methods mentioned earlier. Ethics of care is unique to nursing: other health professions have not taken up the idea of caring as an ethic in itself. More recently, however, the ethics of care approach has been explicitly linked to virtue ethics (van Hooft 1990), suggesting room for further development in terms of knowledge and skills associated with caring, in contrast to the almost exclusive focus so far on personal characteristics and attributes (although this link does depart from the original philosophy behind ethics of care).

Strand 3   Ethics as advocacy

A third strand present in clinical ethics education is ethics as advocacy. This approach to ethics understands the fundamental ethical role of the health professional as being an advocate for the patient (or client). It is founded on the recognition that most healthcare is delivered in a setting where patients are already vulnerable, tend to be rendered voiceless and powerless by the system, and lack knowledge of their options. Advocacy is seen as the everyday ethical remedy for this situation. The knowledge associated with the advocacy strand of ethics teaching is very similar to that in the decision-making strand. In order to advocate for a patient or client, a health professional needs to know what sort of treatment the patient is ethically entitled to, in terms of information, choice, privacy, confidentiality, respect, access to resources and so on. This tends to be expressed in terms of patients' rights rather than principles, but the ethical values grounding both are essentially the same. Hence teaching methods similar to those in the decision-making strand are used. However, the skills and attitudes required for advocacy are arguably quite different from those needed for ethical decision making. An effective advocate has to have courage and resilience, skills in negotiation and putting forward a case, and so on.

Although it could be argued that advocating for patients is part of medical practice, particularly in the context of limitations on resources such as hospital beds and specialist appointments, ethics as advocacy is not a prominent idea in medical ethics education.

The idea of the nurse as patient advocate, however, has a very strong tradition (Thacker 2008, Sorensen & Iedema 2007, Hewitt 2002). Hewitt (2002) describes a number of models of advocacy in nursing that either see advocacy as a natural part of the nurse's role or as a separate task, which requires learning knowledge and skills such as articulating patients' wishes and fostering a patient-centred approach within the health team on behalf of the patient. Both types of advocacy models rely on nurses having the authority, either through their own role in caring for patients or more explicitly as independent advocates, to influence other members of the health team. Writers in this strand acknowledge that, in reality, this can be difficult (Hewitt 2002, Thacker 2008).

Advocacy is also regarded as important in allied health, where it is linked to the nature of the healthcare being provided (Nelson 2005). For example, in social work, advocacy is seen as a primary component of the profession's work (Payne 2005). In a study that examined the moral role of physiotherapists in the United States, advocacy was the characteristic most often identified by participating practitioners (Triezenberg 2005). Advocacy was characterised in that study as a means of broadening the responsibilities of physiotherapist from solely focusing on clinical roles to wider patient management tasks. Similarly, the 2020 vision of the Australian Physiotherapy Association (2005) names advocacy as a key characteristic of future physiotherapists. Its description of advocacy includes contributing effectively to the improved health and wellness of patients and communities; recognising and responding to issues where patients require advocacy; and being an advocate for the physiotherapy profession. The last component highlights links between the concept of advocacy and professional identity or promotion of professionalism as ethical and responsible action. Inclusion of advocacy within allied health ethics curricula means teaching skills of determination (Nelson 2005) and knowledge of the different areas that have the potential to impact on patients, including individuals, organisations and, more broadly, society (Glaser 2005). Despite advocacy skills being discussed as components of good—and by implication, ethical—practice, they tend to be taught as aspirations rather than as specific advocacy skills to enhance ethical practice.

Strand 4   Ethics as moral agency

Concern for moral agency is another strand that is more evident in nursing than in medicine or allied health. Some ethics teaching in nursing focuses on heightening nurses' awareness that they are moral agents, responsible for their own actions and hence needing to make their own ethical decisions, rather than simply having to act on the orders of doctors. This approach to ethics teaching is clearly grounded in long-running tensions between medicine and nursing, and the struggle of nurses to be recognised as autonomous professionals in their own right rather than doctors' handmaidens. Although nursing has come a long way in both theory and practice since the days when nurses were exhorted to simply follow doctors orders' and not think for themselves (Kuhse 1997), nurses still lack decisional authority in the hospital hierarchy.

The moral agency approach to ethics emphasises that nurses are moral agents, not robots, and that many of the ethical dilemmas that they face in practice come from being unable to properly or meaningfully exercise this agency. They are not able to do what they believe is right, or are forced to be involved in practices that they perceive as ethically wrong. The term 'moral distress' has been used commonly within nursing to describe this situation (Jameton 1984, Kalvemark et al 2004). Arguably even worse than the phenomenon of moral distress is the fact that the hierarchical structure of healthcare can destroy or suppress a sense of moral agency altogether. Health professionals with no sense of moral agency do not feel moral distress, as they do not see themselves as doing anything ethically significant or having any decisions to make about how they practise.

In allied health, the idea of moral agency is present, at least implicitly, and is linked to several other strands of ethics education, including the responsibilities associated with being autonomous health professionals, being an advocate for a patient, and being able to justify ethical decisions. For example, the need for therapists to actively reflect on ethical principles, patient perspectives and treatment contexts, is recognised as an expectation of autonomous and ethical practice (Edwards & Delany 2008, Freegard et al 2007). Teaching students to act as moral agents involves assisting them to distinguish between personal and professional values; providing role models and experiences that are likely to extend their opportunity to not only recognise, through case studies and stories, but also participate in actions that require decisions about ethics (Davis 2005, Jensen & Richert 2005).

In medicine, in contrast, ethics as moral agency is not an explicit part of ethics education at all, and is largely not even implicitly present, except perhaps for ethics teaching aimed at medical students in their student role. Medical ethics core curricula tend to reflect the increasing recognition that medical students face a specific set of ethical challenges related to their unique subordinate position in the hospital context (Christakis & Feudtner 1993, Kushner & Thomasma 2001). Issues such as disclosing inexperience, observing seniors' unethical behaviour, and disagreeing with seniors' approach to specific patients arise for medical students: deciding when to speak up is a recurring theme in discussions of these issues. The notion of moral agency is in the background here but rarely receives direct attention. The only other place in medical ethics education where concern about moral agency is implied is in relation to conscientious objection, which medical students are taught is their right in relation to overtly moral matters such as abortion and euthanasia. This sort of right to conscientious objection is also a standard knowledge component of nursing ethics teaching. However, restricting concern about moral agency to specific named moral matters tends to imply that it is not at issue anywhere else. This limits the influence the concept of moral agency might potentially provide in clinical practice.

Although the idea of moral agency is seen as having some importance, especially in nursing, it is not a well-developed ethics teaching practice even there, let alone in allied health or medicine. In teaching terms, the moral agency approach broadly involves encouraging students to recognise their own agency and regard it as important, and empowering them to act as moral agents even in situations of conflict, hierarchical pressures and institutional constraints. This requires ethics education to foster or empower students to develop attitudes of integrity, courage and self worth. However beyond the attitudinal aspect, the more precise knowledge and skills required for moral agency do not receive much attention. Skills and knowledge for ethical decision making are obviously one part of what is needed for moral agency, but are by no means the whole. Skills for getting one's ethical decisions taken seriously by others and acted upon, for example, are also vital. Such skills would encompass clear and persuasive communication underpinned by knowledge of professional roles and responsibilities within different clinical settings.

Strand 5   Ethics as professional identity

The fifth strand present in clinical ethics education as a whole is ethics as professional identity. Professional identity is concerned with the roles, responsibilities, boundaries and overall ethos of a health profession's practice.

The term 'professional behaviour' has two broad meanings (Kerridge et al 2005). The first is as a means of identifying a group of people who are engaged in an occupation with a higher aim or whose work involves acting for the welfare of others. This first meaning is clearly connected to the goals of ethics education. Fullinwider (1996) suggests that professional identity, expressed in terms of specialised knowledge, skills and training, serves to highlight the comparative vulnerability and dependency of patients. It is exposing this power or knowledge differential that provides the motivation and rationale to be concerned with ethics in the first place, and therefore connects the concept of health professional identity with a sense of moral purpose.

The second meaning of professional behaviour used is behaviour that is objective, detached and evidence based. This meaning also provides a rationale for including professional identity in ethics curricula. Knowledge of professional roles and boundaries—such as limits of expertise, recognition of acceptable relationships with colleagues and patients, and an understanding of particular roles within the healthcare team—helps practitioners negotiate ethical dilemmas that involve conflicts in relationships and professional hierarchies. This second rationale is concerned with providing a way of empowering students to better understand and resolve ethical dilemmas related to their professional work.

While the professional identity and ethos of doctors is a recognised component of the medical curriculum (Siegler 2002), it is usually expressed in terms of defining the scope of medical professional practice (Goldie 2000), rather than as an explicit way to empower students to negotiate ethical dilemmas in clinical practice. This is perhaps attributable to the fact that medical practitioners arguably already have a dominant and powerful professional identity in the healthcare team. This strand is therefore seen more strongly in the health professions that have had to devote considerable effort in establishing themselves as independent and worthwhile professions.

In allied health practice, there is a clear connection between having an understanding of one's professional ethos and identity, and having the sense of confidence and ability to address ethical issues in clinical practice (Finch & Geddes 2005, Stiller 2000, Aveyard et al 2005). Allied health ethics education that is directed to this connection focuses on teaching knowledge of expected professional behaviours, including relationships with patients and healthcare colleagues, and professional boundaries and expectations of accountability. Skills that are given attention in this strand of ethics education include being able to articulate and defend one's professional role, knowing how to work with teams of diverse professionals, and how to negotiate healthcare decisions when there is a hierarchy of decision making within the healthcare team.

In nursing, the place of professionalism in ethics is more contestable. In one way, it seems out of place because of the inherent conflict between promoting the detached or objective component of professionalism as a way of defining accountable and ethical practice, and the contrasting view of their professional identity as providing care that is intrinsically ethical (Kerridge et al 2005). However, in another way, it is highly relevant because one of the drivers of a sense of moral agency is an understanding of oneself as a professional. Developing professional identity and autonomy is a strong influence in nursing education, but is not necessarily a strong strand in the ethics curricula.

One way of explaining the development of and different emphases that health professions place on their ethics education, including why some strands are either missing or de-emphasised, is to examine the history and development of the professions. Linker (2005) refers to the early 1900's role of nurses to feed, bathe and cheer recuperating patients. Occupational therapists' role at that time was to nurture 'nervous' patients back to health through simple and non-physically taxing forms of manual labour, so as to pre-occupy their mind and bring about 'psychic well being' (p 329). In contrast, the early work of physiotherapists was portrayed as a career that required athleticism and physical strength. Because physiotherapists sometimes elicited pain to improve health, they did not fit the mould of the 'female professional nurturer'.

Physiotherapy provides one example of the way the history of a profession can influence its understanding and teaching of ethics. In the United States, Australia and United Kingdom, physiotherapists have worked at establishing and maintaining a professional and scientific standard in line with their medical colleagues (Linker 2005, Bentley & Dunstan 2007, Barnitt 1998, Elkin & Anderson 1998). Professional identity has directly influenced the interest in and development of ethics knowledge in the physiotherapy profession. 'The women who drafted the American Physiotherapy Association 1935 code of ethics did not think of themselves as moral philosophers, instead they considered themselves to be masters of a new professional field that needed to be put on firmer ground' (Linker 2005, p 343).

Linker argues, on the basis of this comparative analysis of health professions' professional development, that if care-based service-oriented ethics is the rule among female health professionals, then physiotherapy is the exception to the rule. This provides an explanation for why ethical reasoning and advocacy has developed as a strong strand in physiotherapy ethics literature in contrast to the development of an ethos of caring and virtue in nursing teaching and practice.

An awareness of the origin and development of the different strands, including how and why different health professions have incorporated them into their ethics education, provides many potential advantages for ethics curricula developers. Being in a position to provide students with knowledge of different strands of ethics education, including their associated knowledge, attitudes and skills, potentially enriches students' understanding of the ethics education background of their health professional colleagues. This may lead to enhanced collaboration, tolerance and understanding within the multidisciplinary clinical setting. Second, it allows educators to take a step back and critically review the content and assumptions of the ethics curriculum. There may be historical reasons why some strands are included and others not. But there might also be good pedagogical reasons for changing the focus and mix, even including new strands. By clearly identifying the key elements of each strand, educators are in a better position to develop their own curricula to meet hidden and visible challenges.

The strands and the hidden curriculum

The strands also offer ways of meeting the challenge presented by the 'hidden curriculum'. Regardless of their approach to ethics education, educators inevitably confront this significant barrier in promoting their students' ethical practice as professionals. The hidden curriculum, in our view, constitutes the greatest challenge facing ethics education. Hafferty and Franks articulated the concept of the hidden curriculum in relation to medical education in the mid 1990s, highlighting that '[f]ormal instruction in medical ethics does not take place within a cultural vacuum' (Hafferty & Franks 1994, p 864). They argued that 'medical training at root is a process of moral enculturation' (Hafferty & Franks 1994, p 861) in which informal processes such as observation of doctors' behaviour exercise the greatest influence on students' ethical outlook. Students' role models in the hospitals teach the hidden curriculum, a set of peer-sanctioned values, attitudes and behaviours that may starkly contrast with the content of the formal ethics curriculum students encounter.

Although originally conceptualised in the medical context, the notion of a hidden curriculum seems equally applicable to nursing and allied health professions. While allied health professionals are taught the ethical ideals and principles that form an important component of their future work as independent practitioners, the realities of working (relatively) non-autonomously within multidisciplinary settings, hospital hierarchies and with third party providers in private settings provide a different set of ethical challenges. In nursing, a gap is found between the ideals and theories of caring and nurturing and the reality of working to prove and maintain professionalism and a measure of autonomy in the health system. In each of these disciplines, it is likely that students' experiences in the clinical context powerfully shape their understanding of appropriate behaviour in ways that potentially undermine the efforts of ethics educators.

The hidden curriculum presents an enormous stumbling block for ethics education, but even in medical education, where the phenomenon was first clearly identified, the response has not gone far beyond noticing and deploring its negative effects. Clearly something more positive is required. We suggest several strategies for curriculum developers. First, the issue of the hidden curriculum needs to be highlighted to students within the formal curriculum. Its challenges need to be discussed directly and reflectively with students as part of their formal ethics education. Second, ethics education must equip students to deal with the hidden curriculum in their learning and working environments. To fail to do so is to position students for an inevitable experience of moral distress, where they cannot carry out the actions or manifest the values they have learnt to be morally right. Ethics education that aims to teach the moral role of health practitioners to care for patients, to act in their best interests, to provide the most beneficial care available, and to respect patients' rights, assumes that in practice the practitioner will have the autonomy, authority and resources to undertake such actions (Hewitt 2002, Finch & Geddes 2005, Campbell et al 2007). It is part of ethics educators' duty of care to their students to equip them to deal with the mixed and conflicting messages of the hidden curriculum, and to ensure the assumptions underpinning the ethics program are accurate. Appropriate ethics education needs to be re-conceptualised as education that enables students to recognise and deal effectively with the hidden curriculum.

There are resources within some of the strands discussed earlier that would be helpful here. For example, the moral agency strand, currently of little prominence in ethics curricula (except perhaps in nursing) offers ideas about the knowledge, skills and attitudes that would be helpful in empowering students to engage critically with the hidden curriculum. However, teaching about how to act as a moral agent could move beyond outlining necessary attributes of moral courage, sensitivity, and awareness of professional responsibilities to focus on ways of engaging with aspects of the hidden curriculum that might challenge ideals of moral agency. Teaching students to perceive themselves as moral agents facilitates their appropriate questioning of the ethically problematic modes of practice they observe. In addition to describing attributes of moral agency, students need to be provided with information, theories and research about medical socialisation and professional enculturation, and encouraged to reflect on and develop strategies of communication including conflict negotiation, assertiveness and active engagement with healthcare colleagues and patients.

Similarly, the strands of advocacy and professionalism have the potential to provide practical ways to engage with the hidden curriculum. Although professionalism, and the formal and visible behaviours it encourages, has been criticised as a means to protect particular professional practices and boundaries (Coady & Bloch 1996), there may be value in some of its central tenets that might act to combat the effects of the hidden curriculum. For example, when the professional duty to act objectively, demonstrate respect for the patient and act in their best interests is applied to the challenges posed by the hidden curriculum, the focus of ethics case studies might be directed towards fostering an ability to not only weigh up the relevance and priority of one or more prima facie ethical principles, but also to consider how professionalism should be interpreted and applied when patients are treated unfairly or disrespectfully. In the same way, when advocacy is placed within the context of the hidden curriculum, students will need to be taught interactional skills that not only enable them to recognise and demonstrate respect for a patient's autonomous right to contribute to their healthcare decisions, but they will also need to know how to react to the inevitable times when patients' rights are compromised. Encouraging students, through the use of the agency and advocacy approaches, to see themselves as shaping their working environment has the potential to counter the current tendency towards assimilation at the expense of critical reflection and ethical practice.

The strands that teach ethics as ethical decision making or ethics as a caring attitude provide less practical ways to deal with the hidden curriculum. The caring as ethics strand in particular, is arguably detrimental to successful engagement with the effects of medical socialisation. By an inward focus on developing a particular internal attitude or caring disposition, we argue there is a danger of withdrawing from the discourse of multi-disciplinary practice, diversity and the hidden curriculum. Moreover, promoting an internal dialogue of care may have the effect of facilitating outward displays of professional subordination and maintenance of the hierarchical 'status quo'. Relying exclusively on an ethics of care underpinned by attitudes of virtue and empathy runs counter to the ideals of professionalism, where it is important to not only uphold but also to demonstrate commitment to care, beneficence and respect for patients and colleagues. Finally, the strand of ethics as decision making, while firmly established and grounded in ethical theory and principles, provides an important but arguably abstract way of dealing with the real ethical challenges of clinical practice, that neglects to some extent the influence of healthcare culture, organisational factors, available resources and hierarchies present in healthcare environments.

Each of the five strands discussed in this chapter work individually or in combination towards agreed and established aims of ethics eduction (Goldie 2000): to recognise humanistic aspects of healthcare practice; to encourage an awareness of personal and professional moral commitments; to be able to draw from philosophical, social and legal knowledge in making ethical decisions; and to have appropriate interactional skills to apply the mix of knowledge, attitudes and skills in clinical care. Examining how the strands meet the ethical issues actually encountered in practice and how they work to combat the threats to ethical practice, is an important way in which educators' familiarity with the various strands can enable development of relevant and successful ethics curricula.

Looking to the future, we believe that the fundamental challenge for ethics education is to effectively address the hidden curriculum. While the strands of moral agency and advocacy offer some avenues for curriculum development in the face of the hidden curriculum, we believe that in the first instance focused, education-related research is required. Knowing more about the constituent values of the hidden curriculum in various disciplinary contexts, its effects on students and junior practitioners, and the ways in which healthcare professionals negotiate this set of cultural norms is essential if educators are to be able to design curricula and deliver teaching that meets the challenges posed by the phenomenon. Such information, together with an awareness of the various strands of ethics education and the concepts and resources they offer to both educators and students, will enable educators to design curricula that best equip students to practise well in the ethically complex multidisciplinary environments they encounter as healthcare professionals.

References

Australian Physiotherapy Association 2005 APA Vision for Physiotherapy 2020 Australian Physiotherapy Association. Online. Available: http://physiotherapy.asn.au/index.php/about-the-apa/one-united-voice Accessed 13 Jan 2009

Ashcroft R, Baron D et al 1998 Teaching medical ethics and law within medical education: a model for the UK core curriculum. Journal of Medical Ethics 24(3):188–192

ATEAM 2001 An ethics core curriculum for Australasian medical schools. Medical Journal of Australia 175:205–210

Aveyard H, Edwards S, West S 2005 Core topics of health care ethics: the identification of core topics for interprofessional education. Journal of Interprofessional Care 19(1):63–69

Barnitt R 1998 Ethical dilemmas in occupational therapy and physical therapy: a survey of practitioners in the UK National Health Service. Journal of Medical Ethics 24(3):193–199

Barnitt R, Partridge C 1997 Ethical reasoning in physical therapy and occupational therapy. Physiotherapy Research International 2(3):178–194

Beauchamp T, Childress JF 2001 Principles of biomedical ethics. Oxford University Press, New York

Bentley P, Dunstan D 2007 The path to professionalism: physiotherapy in Australia to the 1980s. Australian Physiotherapy Association, Melbourne

Campbell AV, Chin J, Voo TC 2007 How can we know that ethics education produces ethical doctors? Medical Teacher 29(5):431–436

Chapparo C, Ranker J 2000 Clinical reasoning in occupational therapy. In: Higgs J, Jones M (eds) Clinical reasoning in the health professions, 2nd edn. Butterworth-Heinemann, Oxford

Christakis DA, Feudtner C 1993 Ethics in a short white coat: the ethical dilemmas that medical students confront. Academic Medicine 68(4):249–254

Coady M, Bloch S 1996 Codes of ethics and the professions. Melbourne University Press, Melbourne

Culver C, Clouser K et al 1985 Basic curricular goals in medical ethics. New England Journal of Medicine 312:253–256

Davis C 2005 Educating adult health professionals for moral action: in search of moral courage. In: Purtilo R, Jensen G, Brasic Royeen C (eds) Educating for Moral Action. FA Davis, Philadelphia, p 215–224

Doane G, Pauly B, Brown H et al 2004 Exploring the heart of ethical nursing practice: implications for ethics education. Nursing Ethics 11(3):240–253

Drane JF 1988 Becoming a good doctor: the place of virtue and character in medical ethics. Sheed & Ward, Kansas City

Eaton L, Crotts D, Jensen G 2003 Exploration of ethical decision making in clinical practice: case study comparison of novice and experienced physical therapists. Presented at World Congress of Physical Therapists Conference, Barcelona

Edwards I, Braunack-Mayer A, Jones M 2005 Ethical reasoning as a clinical-reasoning strategy in physiotherapy. Physiotherapy 91:229–236

Edwards I, Delany C 2008 Ethical reasoning. In: Higgs J, Jones M, Loftus S, Christensen N (eds) Clinical reasoning in the health professions, 3rd edn. Elsevier, Boston, p 279–289

Elkin S, Anderson L 1998 Ethics and physiotherapy: an introduction. New Zealand Journal of Physiotherapy Dec:9–18

Finch E, Geddes E 2005 Ethically-based clinical decision making in physical therapy: process and issues. Physiotherapy Theory and Practice 21(3):147–162

Freegard H, Goddard T, Isted L 2007 Human rights and health. In: Freegard H (ed) Ethical practice in health professions. Thomson, Sydney

Fry ST, Johnstone MJ 2002 Ethics in nursing practice: a guide to ethical decision-making, 2nd edn. Blackwell Publishing, Oxford

Fullinwider R 1996 Professional codes and moral understanding. In: Coady M, Glaser J 2005 Three realms of ethics: an integrating map of ethics for the future. In: Purtilo R, Goldie J 2000. Review of ethics curricula in undergraduate medical education, Medical Education 34:108–119

Goldie J 2000 Review of ethics curricula in undergraduate medical education. Medical Education 34:108–119

Hafferty FW, Franks R 1994 The hidden curriculum, ethics teachings and the structure of medical education. Academic Medicine 69(11):861–871

Hewitt J 2002 A critical review of the arguments debating the role of the nurse advocate. Journal of Advanced Nursing 37(5):439–445

Jameton A 1984 Nursing practice: the ethical issues. Prentice-Hall, Englewood Cliffs

Jensen G, Richert A 2005 Reflections on the teaching of ethics in physical therapist education: integrating cases, theory and learning. Journal of Physical Therapy Education 19:78–85

Kalvemark S, Hoglund A, Hansson M, Westerholm P, Arnetz B 2004 Living with conflicts: ethical dilemmas and moral distress in the health care system. Social Science & Medicine, 58:1075–1084

Kenny B, Lincoln M, Balandin S 2007 A dynamic model of ethical reasoning in speech pathology. Journal of Medical Ethics 33:508–513

Kerridge I, Lowe M, McPhee J 2005 Ethics and law for the health professions, 2nd edn. Federation Press, Sydney

Kuhse H 1997 Caring: nurses, women and ethics. Blackwell, Oxford

Kushner TK, Thomasma DC (eds) 2001 Ward ethies: dilemmas for medical students and doctors in training. Cambridge University Press, UK

Leininger M, McFarland M 1995 Transcultural nursing: concepts, theories, research and practice. McGraw-Hill, New York

Linker B 2005 The business of ethics: gender, medicine, and the professional codification of the American Physiotherapy Association, 1918–1935. Journal of the History of Medicine 60:320–354

Nelson L 2005 Professional responsibility and advocacy for access to rehabilitation services: a case study in lymphedema services in Vermont. In: Purtilo R, Jensen G, Brasic Royeen C (eds) Educating for moral action, EA Davis, Philadelphia

Oakley J, Cocking D 2001 Virtue ethics and professional roles. Cambridge University Press, UK

Payne M 2005 Modern social work theory, 3rd edn. Lyceum Books, Chicago

Pellegrino ED, Thomasma DC 1993 The virtues in medical practice. Oxford University Press, New York

Peloquin S 2005 Affirming empathy as a moral disposition. In: Purtilo R, Jensen G, Brasic Royeen C (eds) Educating for moral action. FA Davis, Philadelphia

Poulis I 2007 Bioethics and physiotherapy. Journal of Medical Ethics (33):435–436

Purtilo R 1999 Ethical dimensions in the health professions, 3rd edn. WB Saunders, Philadelphia

Purtilo R 2005 Ethical dimensions in the health professions, 4th edn. Elsevier Saunders, Philadelphia

Rogers S 2005 Portrait of occupational therapy. Journal of Interprofessional Care 19(1):70–79

Siegler M 2002 Training doctors for professionalism: some lessons from teaching clinical medical ethics. Mount Sinai Journal of Medicine 69:404–409

Sorensen R, Iedema R 2007 Advocacy at end-of-life: research design: an ethnographic study of an ICU. International Journal of Nursing Studies 44(8):1343–1353

Stiller C 2000 Exploring the ethos of the physical therapy profession in the United States: social, cultural, and historical influences and their relationship to education. Journal of Physical Therapy Education 14(3):7–15

Thacker KS 2008 Nurses' advocacy behaviours in end-of-life nursing care. Nursing Ethics 15(2):174–185

Thompson I, Melia K, Boyd K 2000 Nursing ethics, 4th edn. Churchill Livingstone, Edinburgh

Triezenberg H 2005 Examining the moral role of physical therapists. In: Purtilo R, Jensen G, Brasic Royeen C (eds) Educating for moral action. EA Davis, Philadelphia

van Hooft S 1990 Moral education for nursing decisions. Journal of Advanced Nursing 15:210–215

van Hooft S, Gillam L, Byrnes M 1995 Facts and values: an introduction to critical thinking for nurses. MacLennan & Petty, Sydney

Vanlaere L, Gastmans C 2007 Ethics in nursing education: learning to reflect on care practices. Nursing Ethics 14(6):759–766

Watson J 1979 Nursing: the philosophy and science of caring. Little Brown, Boston

Index

➡